The Consumer Handbook on Hearing Loss and Hearing Aids

A Bridge to Healing

2nd Edition

**CHAPTERS RECOMMENDED BY YOUR
H   VIDER**

Dedication

To you with courage to seek change. . .

The Consumer Handbook on Hearing Loss and Hearing Aids

A Bridge to Healing

2nd Edition

Edited by
Richard Carmen, Au.D.
Doctor of Audiology

Auricle Ink Publishers • Sedona Arizona

Library of Congress Cataloging-in-Publication Data

The consumer handbook on hearing loss and hearing aids : a bridge to healing / edited by Richard Carmen.-- 2nd ed.
  p. cm.
Includes bibliographical references and index.
  ISBN 0-9661826-2-6 (hbk.) -- ISBN 0-9661826-1-8 (pbk.)
1. Deafness--Handbooks, manuals, etc. 2. Hearing disorders--Handbooks, manuals, etc. 3. Hearing aids--Handbooks, manuals, etc. 4. Hearing impaired--Rehabilitation--Handbooks, manuals, etc. I. Carmen, Richard.

RF290.C665 2004
617.8'9--dc22

2003020383

©2004 by Auricle Ink Publishers

First Printing

ISBN 0-9661826-1-8 (Soft Cover)
ISBN 0-9661826-2-6 (Hard Cover)

Cover Concept and Development by Jane Pirini

This book is available at special discount when ordered in bulk quantities. Contact the publisher for more information.

Auricle Ink Publishers
P.O. Box 20607, Sedona AZ 86341
Tel (928) 284-0860
Fax (928) 284-2370
www.hearingproblems.com
E-mail: AIP@hearingproblems.com

TABLE OF CONTENTS

Introduction
Douglas L. Beck, Au.D.

Dr. Beck received his Doctor of Audiology Degree from the University of Florida, and currently resides in San Antonio, Texas. He has been practicing audiology for 20 years. Dr. Beck is President and Editor-In-Chief of the world's largest professional website for hearing healthcare professionals, www.audiologyonline.com and the most "linked to" hearing healthcare website for consumers and their families, www.healthyhearing.com.

I was deeply honored by Dr. Carmen's invitation to prepare an Introduction to the Second Edition of this wonderful book. I have given patients and their families many copies of the First Edition, so I am quite familiar with it.

Throughout this Second Edition, I was impressed with the content, style and ease with which complicated information is transferred to those with hearing loss and their loved ones. It is a pragmatic approach to improving your quality of life and getting results if you have hearing loss. Day-to-day issues are competently addressed in simple, non-technical language.

The roster of contributors to this book includes some of the most distinguished practitioners in our profession. If you are new to hearing loss issues, hearing aids, or are an experienced hearing aid wearer, you'll find many valuable tips and tremendous guidance through the wealth of knowledge and experience offered by these contributors.

I believe this book will be the single most important educational tool you will discover in your search for better hearing! Those with a desire to seek positive changes and improve their quality of life (and the lives of their loved ones) can do so with the tools found in this book. Between the covers you'll find the inside story from the experts. They'll tell you how to maximize adjustment to hearing loss and how to most benefit from hearing aids. You'll learn who to consult, how to interpret your audiogram, and how to confront deep feelings about hearing loss. You'll read about technology breakthroughs and cutting edge science that will enrich your life. And you'll learn of some challenges that must be endured. Ultimately, you'll be able to assess your level of readiness for help, and most importantly, learn what action you can take to dramatically improve the quality of your life.

If you're a senior, you have certain requirements that come with age which deserve the attention of patient healthcare professionals. You'll learn how to identify these needs so you can remain watchful over them.

While this book can be read cover to cover, it's intended as a *handbook* from which you can pick and choose chapters and sections you find most beneficial. However you use this book, I think you'll find it to be of exceptional benefit.

Congratulations to Dr. Carmen for this wonderful gift to you, and congratulations to you for seeking a better quality of life through knowledge and perseverance.

—*Dr. Douglas L. Beck*

CHAPTER ONE
The Emotions of Losing Hearing and A Bridge To Healing

Richard Carmen, Au.D.

Dr. Carmen received his Doctor of Audiology Degree from the Arizona School of Health Sciences, a division of the Kirksville College of Osteopathic Medicine. He has been practicing audiology and issuing hearing aids since 1972, during which time he pioneered research into the effects of metabolic diseases on hearing. He has written extensively in the field as a regular contributor to various hearing journals, and authored two previous consumer books. His material has appeared in such popular consumer-based periodicals as *The Saturday Evening Post, Ladies' Home Journal* and *Self Magazine*. He currently resides in Sedona Arizona where he manages his clinical practice.

As Quasimodo, the Hunchback of Notre Dame, lay dying in the arms of the beautiful gypsy girl La Esmeralda, a tear rolls down his cheek. On his dying breath, he realizes his greatest torment— the pain of feeling. He whispers to Esmeralda, "Why could I not have been made of stone?"

There is nothing wrong with feeling emotions. After all, they are what characterize us as human. Emotional experiences may be wonderful, painful, and sometimes perplexing. Yet, more than our physical body, feelings are the substance of our identity. Each of us reacts differently toward the varied experiences of our lives. For centuries, fields of study have been devoted to exploring this fascinating phenomenon, but the search seems to have yielded as much controversy as knowledge.

From more than three decades of clinical practice, I've observed some compelling emotions and feelings in my patients. These observations extend into my own family members with loss of hearing, so the feelings we'll be talking about touch home.

I taught an audiology course once in which I had my students wear earplugs for a full day—morning to bedtime. They were asked to log their feelings and emotions and report to the class the following week. We were all overwhelmed by two things: the similarity of their experiences and the depth of their emotions.

Students reported that they felt inadequate and incompetent. There was also a sense of limitation in areas they'd taken for granted. Simple tasks like using the telephone couldn't be performed without special focus, difficulty or strain. Common sounds like ice stirred in a glass, running water or turning a page in a book—sounds that orient us in our environment—suddenly vanished.

Driving the car was a new experience. With the absence of wind and traffic, there was a feeling of disorientation. Students quickly realized how important their vision became to compensate for what they could not hear. Yet, such compensation wasn't enough.

By the end of the day most of the students confessed they were worn out and disturbed by what they had gone through.

"What a horrible experience!" one student remarked.

An apt description I thought.

One student reported she had collapsed into bed crying. Others were unnerved or depressed. Their collective reactions were directly linked to feelings of inadequacy—a deficiency in their daily performance relative to how they were accustomed to functioning. Once the earplugs were removed, all ill feelings dissipated. Their sense of normalcy and calm had returned. If your significant other has no idea what it feels like to have a hearing loss, this might be an enlightening experience.

While this experiment was useful to normal hearing students, it revealed what you no doubt already know. Hearing is an essential human sense. Its absence would be greatly missed by anyone. And as hearing declines, similar to other sensory deficits, we humans have an extraordinary ability to compensate for the loss. Such compensation is a built-in defense mechanism that we give little thought to. It just happens. If you have a heart attack, the body works quickly to establish other arteries and connections. If you lose your sense of smell, your eyes become more probing. If vision goes, hearing usually sharpens. And when hearing deteriorates, an array of latent abilities kick in. When they do, the act of compensation can fool you. You may do well for a while with partial hearing loss, and not even recognize its presence. For example, you might cast it off as poor attention. It's for this reason that loss of hearing gives the impression of being so insidious.

"It just kind of crept up on me!" most hard of hearing people confess. Of course it didn't really just creep up. It's more that early suspicions went ignored.

Something you've probably said many times in your life, and will see repeated, rephrased and re-analyzed in this book is the complaint, "I hear but I don't understand the words clearly!" This is particularly true when trying to communicate in a group, around a few people, or in an environment with background noise such as in a restaurant or automobile. Early on, when you had problems hearing, you may have passed it off as being no more troublesome for you than for anyone else in the same situation. But as issues around poor hearing grew more apparent and the process of communication began breaking down, you must have realized the problem was not going away.

People who develop hearing loss from an explosion, accident, or other physical trauma are probably more inclined to deal with it because it is sudden and readily apparent. But if you're in generally good health and are the type of person who doesn't like to think of yourself as less capable than anyone else, you may have started blaming other people for frequent miscommunication. Typically, you may think others are not speaking clearly or loudly enough, or they "mumble" their words. It's only when sufficient numbers of people close to you suggest that it's you and not them, you usually get your first inkling of something within your personal communication system has gone awry. Some people never come to this realization and go on believing that others are the source of their communication failure. They continue to blame and are discouraged that other people do not enunciate well. This is not healthy for anyone, and why it's so important to address the core issue.

Our ego is attached to our health. We like to think of ourselves as being in shape, with a good heart, teeth, bones, vision, and good hearing. To resist the reality of having hearing loss perpetuates miscommunication and the emotions that go with it. If we try to ignore it, or stop thinking about it, the problem persists. For some people, the crossroads for acknowledging hearing difficulty and doing something about is where they get stuck, and end up doing nothing. In fact, the odds are high that prior to reading this book you've known of your hearing loss for longer than seven years. In the meantime, what problems you thought you had may now be compounded.

Problem-Solving Ground Rules

Before we discuss feelings you may hold surrounding your hearing loss, let's first define the terms used and establish the ground rules upon which problems can be solved. A "hearing loss" is the physical condition in your ear. "Hearing difficulties" pertain to specific situations (like trying to hear someone speaking to you). A "hearing problem" is your internalization, how you process the issues surrounding these situations (like getting upset at your spouse if you miss a word).

These terms are often mistakenly interchanged. If you're in the living room watching television with your family and you realize that you're missing too much dialogue, you might ask others in the room if you can turn the volume louder, in which case you think you've solved the hearing difficulty. The reality is that inevitably your family will object to having the television too loud. This may make you angry, resentful, embarrassed, guilty, selfish, annoyed or other ill feelings—and it's a sure sign of a hearing problem. You're internalizing feelings about a hearing difficulty. As stated earlier, the first step in solving difficulties about your experience is to first acknowledge the difficulty, then recognize how you feel about your hearing loss. A willingness to consider it a fact of life will create a solid bridge to healing. This is the foundation upon which all hearing problems will find resolution.

There are two common philosophies people seem to adopt once hearing loss becomes a part of their lives: you can try to cover up the fact that you have it, or tell others when the occasion is appropriate that you don't hear well. There are many variations between both themes but if you look at yourself honestly, you'll recognize that you are more polarized one way.

The emotions a person feels when hearing loss is confirmed takes the full gamut of human experiences. Some are relieved that at last they know that this is the cause of their problem. Others are horrified—it seems an unbelievable possibility that the problem could be wholly theirs. So many of us react in so many different ways, and each of us seems to have our own specific internal (feelings) and external (people around us) influences, that predicting how we might experience hearing loss becomes quite complex.

Furthermore, your reactions to hearing loss do not necessarily equate to the degree of impairment; that is, you can have a mild loss of hearing which impacts your life more profoundly than someone with greater loss. Your reactions will be most influenced by how you feel about yourself and the world around you, the personality type you're born with, and how other people close to you feel about your problem (or who you've alienated in the process). The most important ground rule to bear in mind when looking at your issues as we progress through this chapter is: *be honest with yourself!*

Self Inquiry

Any problem can have at least two solutions that bring about healing: (1) change the situation, or (2) change how you feel, interact or react. The problem with *changing the situation*, if you're an unaided person with hearing loss, is that you could find yourself continually changing your environment and still not hearing. You may also try to change the environment to avoid an unpleasant experience but it doesn't necessarily help you hear better.

The problem with *changing how you feel* is that it's an imposing challenge. It's very difficult to transform anger into love, frustration into understanding, or embarrassment into delight. Surely, it would seem that it doesn't happen quickly if at all. But I can tell you that it does happen. When people move past whatever has been holding them back from hearing aids, and they finally wear them, not only has a change occurred but how they feel about it becomes apparent to most people in their lives.

The definition of "change" is "giving up something for something else." The difficulty for anyone in making changes is that it requires giving up something to which we've grown accustomed. It is less certain, and sometimes frighteningly unfamiliar. I've always thought that there should be a course teaching students during their first year of college how to gracefully make changes in their lives. How better adjusted to life's experiences we'd all be.

Most of us find we're not skilled in making changes. It's usually something we find uncomfortable. Even good changes are known to cause stress. A move to a better house, getting a higher paying job, or even winning the lottery cause high stress. We tend to want to stick to "the familiar." Yet, going from dysfunction to adjustment necessitates change. To avoid stress, most of us unknowingly tend to stick to bad situations.

Perception has everything to do with the degree of adjustment, acceptance and solutions you embrace with regard to your hearing loss. Many people with hearing loss report they have altered their view of the world around them in an unhealthy way. People who were once soft spoken and gentle sometimes become outspoken and annoyed; others who were once alive with spirit and energy may grow pensive and withdrawn. Those close to them notice these changes and are saddened by it. If you aren't aware of such changes, if in fact they exist, it could be because they usually develop slowly over a period of years.

If you have the courage to really look at the impact hearing loss has had in your life, the following exercise may prove to be revealing. When completed, read the same list to someone who knows you well (your spouse, a grown child or a close friend) and ask this person to respond *how he or she believes you operate in the world.*

Exercise #1

If the statements feel mostly accurate write True; if they feel mostly inaccurate write False:

1) _____ I don't hear well because other people mumble, don't enunciate clearly enough, or talk too low or softly for me to hear.

2) _____ Since I've had this hearing loss, I can't do all the things I'd like to do.

3) _____ People don't dare make jokes about my hearing trouble in my presence.

4) _____ I don't mingle with as many people (old and/or new acquaintances) as I used to because I don't hear well.

5) _____ I just can't be seen wearing a hearing aid.

6) _____ If I'm left alone in a conversation, I don't understand or trust what I hear.

7) _____ I know people think I'm not as sharp as I used to be because I don't hear as well as I once did.

8) _____ If I don't want to hear what someone says the first time, I'll remain quiet; it's a waste of my time trying to hear.

9) _____ I just can't seem to assert myself the way I used to (or as others do) since I lost my ability to hear well.

10)_____ It's difficult for me to accept that I actually have a hearing loss.

11)_____ I recognize that I'm the source of the problem because of my hearing loss; when I miss what somebody says to me, it's not their fault.

12)_____ Even though I have a hearing loss, I still do all the things I used to do.

13) _____ I have humorous things happen to me as a result of my not hearing well.

14) _____ In spite of my hearing loss, I'm careful not to give up any relationships I have in my life, or lose out on any potential relationships, by staying home too much.

15) _____ I would not think of hiding the fact that I was wearing a hearing aid.

16) _____ I feel completely at ease communicating with anyone in most environments even though I have hearing loss.

17) _____ Despite my hearing loss, other people do not think less of me than before my loss developed.

18) _____ I don't mind asking people to repeat what was said if I haven't heard it.

19) _____ As my hearing loss has developed, I have made a systematic effort to compensate for it by being more outgoing.

20) _____ It's easy for me to think of myself as having a hearing loss.

Note: Before you read the following interpretation which will give away the design of this exercise, be sure you and your partner complete it fully.

Interpretation

Statements 1 through 10 are the reverse of 11 through 20, respectively. For example, statement 3 is opposite to statement 13. There are two built-in veracity checks: one is that however you responded to a particular statement, if you're honest with yourself, you should have responded opposite to its corresponding statement. The other check is the way in which your partner responded.

Did you respond consistently to both sides of the statements, True on one, False on the other? Did your partner agree with you? If not, you may want to look carefully at the content of those statements. Are you procrastinating? Do you spend a lot of time with negative thinking about the loss? Are you blaming others?

Or is your outlook healthy? Do you tend to think more positively in handling your hearing loss? Do you try and find the lighter side? Are you just as engaged in life as before you developed loss of hearing?

Once you've examined the way you and your partner responded to the same statements, you may well find that you are the one person who has prevented finding your own solutions. This exercise was not an attempt to change who you are, but rather to *change and improve how you react in the world.*

Denying Hearing Loss

If your hearing healthcare provider informs you that you have an irreversible sensorineural hearing loss, despite the fact that more than 28 million other Americans have it, this is not welcomed news. However, it is quite another story if you don't believe it or choose to do nothing about it.

Most standard dictionaries define *denial* as *the refusal to believe* or *the act of disowning.* It is rejection of the notion that your hearing is an issue. This being so, you not only disown the condition, you decline help because logic dictates that you cannot seek help for something that does not exist:

- "Nobody hears everything!"
- "Don't talk to me from another room and I hear great!"
- "It doesn't bother me!"
- "I just ask people to speak up!"
- "Only my wife (or husband) complains about it!"
- "I ignore it!"

Often, early denial provides a useful function by allowing people time to recover from the initial shock of knowing they have a hearing loss. But some trap themselves here for years. To deny the notion of hearing loss is to claim that you hear well. Denial is the ultimate deception to oneself.

Mechanisms of denial can become an integral part of the way people operate in the world. The more sophisticated and highly developed their compensatory responses, the easier it may be to deny the problem. For example, they may have others help them hear, like asking others to repeat, rephrase, speak up and so forth. Without realizing it, they may even grow skilled at favoring an ear, tuning one person in and another out, repeating what they think they hear to confirm its accuracy, reducing background noises, making educated guesses, watching facial movements and expressions as well as gestures and body language. These are all excellent and necessary ways to hear and understand better, but the irony is people can get stuck believing all of this will solve their problem, and it doesn't.

If you're wondering if you're experiencing denial as you read this book, likely not. If you were in true denial, you probably wouldn't have picked up this book (although you could read it and say, "That's not me he's talking about!"). If you're well aware of the loss, but deny its presence when others inquire, this isn't denial. It's concealment. So, congratulations! At least you're willing to look at the problem. This is where we must begin.

It's been said that uncorrected hearing loss is more noticeable than hearing aids because the act of concealing a hearing loss is doomed to fail. It can make a person appear foolish, inattentive, disinterested, confused, senile or mentally challenged. A person operating at this level needs to understand the serious emotional hardships imposed on oneself, the spouse, family and friends. Denying or minimizing the impact the loss has in one's life (or in the life of others) does not solve the problem. Having others "hear" for you is not the answer either. In fact, these things compound the problem in close relationships. "Why should I carry the burden?" an honest but resentful spouse asks!

You might feel annoyed that you have a hearing loss but your spouse is annoyed that you do nothing about it. You may isolate yourself from family gatherings because you can't hear, or feel foolish, or get embarrassed, but your family feels abandoned and dismissed that they aren't important enough to you. Your unwillingness to seek help can create the feeling in loved ones and friends that you are selfish or irresponsible.

Procrastination

Something that may have tended to fool you is that sometimes you hear beautifully, other times poorly. Loved ones may also observe this to be true. This gives the false impression that you have a *listening issue*, not a hearing problem. This is the elusive nature of the condition for many people. You may believe room acoustics are the problem, or that it's other people—they talk like they have marbles in their mouth or "mumble." You may hear people differently because some voices project better than others. Men are usually easier to hear than women or children. And the environment plays a significant role. The bottom line is that the configuration of loss you have may allow you to hear some voices well, others poorly.

Putting off the hearing evaluation (or hearing aids) can be based on what seems like valid logic:

- "I'm too young!"
- "It's not bad enough yet!"
- "No one I know likes their hearing aids!"

- "We just can't afford it now!"
- "After we paint the house!"
- "Tom has a hearing loss and doesn't wear hearing aids and he gets along just fine!" (but of course Tom really doesn't).

Such people recognize the presence of the loss but try to find every excuse not to do anything about it. This is procrastination. In the presence of other health concerns, this may seem like just one more issue you may or may not eventually get to. However, in the absence of any other health problems, hearing loss may not seem important enough to address:

- After I do my teeth!"
- I don't want to spend my children's inheritance!"
- If only Medicare paid for it!"
- It's that trip to Hawaii (a new car, a child's wedding) or hearing aids!"

Any of this sound familiar? If so, it's worth reading further to explore this more thoroughly. Just buckle your seatbelt.

Emotions Behind Hearing Loss

How you deal with hearing loss is probably how you deal with life. We all develop patterns by three to five years of age by which time they become entrenched in our personality. While you may wish to act and react differently, to a certain extent, it means deprogramming yourself. Despite such imposing challenges against change, to attempt change precludes the *desire* or *intent* to change. As you are about to discover, failure to change by not seeking help for your hearing loss is now linked to a myriad of emotional problems, some permanent, but most preventable.

As you explore your internal emotional processes, if you feel you don't deal with them in the way you would like, you would be well advised (individually or as a couple) to consider consulting a psychotherapist. I am not suggesting long-term therapy, but a few sessions where an unbiased, arbitrary, properly trained therapist can act as your personal sounding board. This can prove to be a very rewarding, productive and nurturing experience.

The Effects of Sensory Deprivation

Sensory deprivation research was popular in the 1950s and told us much about the human experience in the absence of stimulation. John Lilly, MD[1] authored a few pop culture books on this subject matter, as well as scientific papers that were informative and fascinating. He was the creator of the "Lilly Tank," where one floated on Epson salts sealed inside a tank, had no body awareness, no light and no sound.

As auditory, visual and sensual input diminishes with less stimulation to corresponding neural centers in the brain, the brain is not happy. Lilly's students subjected to these experiments generally could not tolerate the absence of sensory stimulation longer than a few hours or a few days. Besides altered realities, other complaints included feelings of disorientation and inability to concentrate. You should know that people who suffer from hearing loss (which is auditory deprivation) also report *the same symptoms.*

Solitary confinement in prisons is sensory deprivation to the extreme. Over time, it has been shown to cause permanent problems, most profoundly, *intolerance to social interaction.* Obviously, this effect is counterproductive to a society that desires paroled inmates to be re-acclimated into society. By no coincidence, symptoms found among many people with untreated hearing loss (auditory deprivation) also include *intolerance to social interaction.*

Much of reality (what little we understand of it) is based on our very delicate sensory systems. Impairment to any one of our five senses *does result in an altered state of reality.* If you miss portions of communication and perhaps do not realize it, you are experiencing one thing while something else entirely may have been intended. When you experience auditory deprivation, your natural instinct is to avoid social situations because just like students in Lilly's experiments, not many people like living in an altered state of reality.

Furthermore, there is now reliable scientific evidence to document the fact that untreated hearing loss can lead to a variety of unhealthy emotional conditions. The Hearing Instrument Association in conjunction with the National Council on Aging ran a study with over 2,000 hard of hearing adults and over 1700 family members.[2] (Dr. Kochkin will discuss this further in Chapter 4.)

This study concluded that people who suffer from hearing loss were more likely to experience increased anger, frustration, paranoia, insecurity, instability, nervousness, tension, anxiety, irritability, discontentment, depression, being temperamental, fearful, more likely to be self-critical, suffer from a sense of inferiority, social phobias, be perceived as confused, disoriented or unable to concentrate. Experiencing only one of these would seem enough to inspire one to seek help, but unfortunately, many people with hearing loss tend to experience a variety of these unhealthy emotional states.

In addition, research has shown that failure to stimulate hearing (the auditory portion of the brain) by not wearing hearing aids may result in a more rapid decline in speech recognition.[3-4] These reports were based on a substantial number of subjects who possessed at least a moderate degree of hearing loss in both ears but received only one hearing aid. As a result of auditory deprivation in the unaided ear, a reduction in speech recognition occurred. In some cases, this was reversible by adding a second hearing aid.

If hearing loss is not addressed as a major health issue, the risks of negative emotional impact are far too great. These are consequences that can be avoided, but often are not because people do not realize the influence of untreated hearing loss. What follows will give you a sense of this impact.

Isolation, Avoidance, Anxiety & Social Phobias

As we age and begin to lose longtime friends and loved ones, we find ourselves more isolated. Impaired hearing only adds to this isolation, and compounds matters. The experience of separation from others is not limited to the over-fifty crowd. Many patients in their twenties and thirties give up their favorite activities because of their inability to hear adequately. I've seen high school students refuse to wear hearing aids because they feared peer ridicule. They sadly preferred to be left alone and miss out on social interaction than risk being seen wearing hearing aids.

Social phobias can and do commonly develop from untreated hearing loss.[5] A social phobia is a form of anxiety; a persistent fear of social or performance situations in which embarrassment may occur. For example, if you avoided a particular social obligation with your significant other because you feared the embarrassing consequences of your hearing loss, and these types of things were persistent and excessive for more than six months, you would have a diagnosable social phobia.

If you have noticed that you've been avoiding social situations as described, you have reason to be concerned. Fundamentally, you're cutting yourself off from the very nurturing people who make you feel loved in the world. Clearly not a healthy choice. Apart from hearing loss, these anxiety disorders are serious medical conditions affecting more than 19 million American adults and can grow progressively worse if untreated. Through the 1990s, anxiety disorders in the U.S. grew by more than 50 percent and now pose a major public health concern. Interestingly, according to the National Institute on Deafness and Other Communication Disorders (NIDCD), hearing loss is the third most prevalent chronic condition in older Americans. So, if you're an older American experiencing hearing loss, you have much greater risk for isolation and avoidance of common pleasures in life.

Depression

More than 22 percent of Americans ages 18 and older suffer from a diagnosable mental disorder in a given year,[6] and major depressive disorder is the leading cause of disability in the U.S. and established market economies worldwide.[7] The average age of onset is in the twenties with twice as many women as men affected by depressive disorders. A fact you should know is that those who suffer from hearing loss have a greater likelihood of also suffering from depression.[8]

These are staggering statistics. Despite these facts, depression is *not* a natural part of aging. It can be prevented, and is treatable in about 80 percent of older adults. A major source of depression, especially in older adults, can be untreated hearing loss. The simple action of wearing hearing aids can resolve depression associated with untreated hearing loss. In older adults, this should be pursued aggressively, since depression is also commonly associated with anxiety and other simultaneously occurring ailments. As we age, our normal coping abilities diminish. It is so important to restore as much normal functioning as we can, at any age, but especially in these later years.

So often we think that what we feel inside remains hidden there. It's easy to forget that those we love can usually see past this thin veil of illusion. And rest assured, if depression is there, they'll eventually see it, and no doubt be suffering right along with you.

Anger

Anger is a kind of stepchild to depression. In clinical terms, anger is often described as *depression turned inward.* When left untreated, people with depression can be difficult to be around, but something you may be surprised to hear is that you have a right to be angry! It's your body. Hearing is a needed and vital sense. Its loss influences almost every aspect of socialization. Every time you ask people to repeat themselves, it's a quiet reminder of a problem that does not go away.

The problem with anger is that it typically finds its vent outwardly. Eventually, you can become resentful and angry at others over your own need to have things repeated. Worse yet, you may become angry when a family member suggests you should get help. You already know that, you just don't want to hear it from anyone. For some, it's just too painful.

The dynamics of this emotion can be fairly simple. You become angry that you're not hearing. The family is upset that this "stubborn person" isn't doing more about the hearing loss. Some hard of hearing people, oblivious to the impact their hearing loss has on others, may ask to have things repeated in a blaming manner. This leads others to feel that the communication problem extends *to them,* and therefore gets them angry!

If you recognize that anger is an issue for you, you may find that you're as angry with the world as you are with yourself. Perhaps you desperately want to make a change but don't know how or where to turn. Indecision can keep you angry and upset. If you continue ignoring the problem, the issues surrounding it are further perpetuated. If you find solace in reverting to denial of the problem, it's a reprieve—but short-lived—you've already awakened to the truth of your situation.

For most people, unexpressed inner turmoil finally shifts from its simmering, hidden view, to boiling over. People around you are less likely to understand from where this hostility arises if you yourself are not in touch with it. You risk friends and family support diminishing as rapidly as your quality of life.

Once you become attuned that your upset originates from how you feel about yourself (that is, the anger that you carry because of what hearing loss has done to your life), and are willing to do something about it, you may discover a renewed sense of calm.

Selfishness and Resentment

Living with someone who refuses to get help, regardless of the condition, is a challenge. But coming to terms with hearing loss can be a very slow journey for many. If you expect others to compensate for your loss of hearing instead of assuming this responsibility yourself, you could be setting up a fertile environment for strained family relationships. Your negligence may rightfully be seen as a selfish act. Of course you're entitled to expect others not to speak to you from another room, or in the presence of such cacophony as a loud television, a vacuum cleaner or music. But in the absence of wearing hearing aids, the family shouldn't be expected to manipulate the household for your convenience, especially when it's at the expense of others you care about.

If you're out socially and you're unaided, you already know how fed up your friends and loved ones are over seeing you miss out on conversation. If you're in a movie theater (if in fact you're not avoiding theaters altogether) and your spouse or friend must continuously repeat the on-screen dialogue, you might be hearing a lot of, "Shhh!" from those seated near you. In the meantime, you, your partner and maybe others around you have just missed another line of dialogue.

Frustration and Defeat

In any family where a member has hearing loss, you'll find frustration. For someone who doesn't have hearing loss, it's almost impossible to conceptualize the depth of this problem. After all, there's no physical sign—no bandages on the head, no fractured bones, no walker. Because you give the general appearance of looking so normal, others may expect you to *hear normally*. Your spouse may continue to talk to you from other rooms, or with a back turned or with a pencil in the mouth.

Worse, you tell your physician that you believe you have a hearing loss and are surprised what you're told. Research has shown that, first, your physician will not test you nor will he or she likely refer you. To add insult to injury, you are probably told: "Don't worry about it. Everyone eventually has some. I have a little myself but I just ignore it!" If your physician has told you ignore it, it is well meant but incorrect and misguided information that will merely add to your mounting frustrations. You should know you are not alone. Eighty-six percent of doctors in the U.S. still *do not* screen for hearing loss![9]

Early in your experience of hearing loss you may have actually laughed at many of the misheard words. I was with my wife at the hardware store when I thought I heard her say, "Do you need some *coffee?*"

I was insulted because I took it to mean she thought I was not paying attention, but she had said, "Do you need some *caulking!*"

Another time when I asked my wife about what I should wear to a particular party, she said, "Leave your clothes!" Hardly, I thought! I only heard it correctly when she repeated it. "*Leisure* clothes!" Good thing she repeated it!

Worse yet is when you think you hear everything quite clearly but none of it makes sense, perhaps mixed with other thoughts you heard perfectly. Repeating doesn't help because with a hearing loss at specific frequencies, the same words are generated at the same frequencies you do not hear well.

My 7-year-old daughter was in the backseat of the car and hollered up front, "Daddy, did you see my new *minty mouth wash?*"

Now that made perfect sense to me, but when I told her she had to keep it in her bathroom cabinet, not laying around the counter, she was dumbfounded. "Why would I do that?" she asked.

"Because that's where minty mouth wash belongs!"

"Dad! I didn't say my minty mouth wash. I said *Mickey Mouse Watch!*"

Over time, the humor of mistakes seems to dwindle. What remains are still day-to-day frustrations. Eventually, it can lead to a culmination of mixed emotions as we've discussed, especially annoyance and anger fueled by frustrations.

A frequently heard comment by the person with hearing loss, as well as the family, is, "I can't stand it anymore!" In fact, the longer untreated hearing loss persists, the greater the frustrations for everyone.

In addition to frustration, it's easy to feel defeated and not know what else to do. You struggle to hear despite how attentive you are. You're playing an odds game—sooner or later you're going to miss some conversation. Defeat could be your fate if there was no help available. Not taking advantage of professional help is not defeat, *it's self-defeat*. It is resignation, concession, submission and surrender. It does nothing to lessen the problem. (If you already wear hearing aids and feel defeated, explore all other options available to you, *many included in this book*.)

Embarrassment

Of the array of emotions you can go through with loss of hearing, something common to everyone is embarrassment. Second-guessing what you think you hear, offering inappropriate responses, missing the punch line to a joke, or getting wrong directions are small examples of what you and loved ones experience. If you're not comfortable with your communication skills, your subtle cues of awkwardness will put others ill at ease.

People often do not pursue help for themselves because the thought of wearing hearing aids is embarrassing. Ironically, failure to do so usually proves to be more embarrassing. With the advent of the CIC (completely-in-the-canal) hearing aids in the early 1990s, this trend has shifted. The cosmetic appeal of these exceptionally inconspicuous hearing aids have attracted wearers who would never have considered amplification on any other basis.

Hopefully, with continuing technology, embarrassment about hearing aid use will become a thing of the past. In the hearing healthcare world of today, hearing aids and other appropriate amplification accessories offer anyone with loss of hearing the most efficient avenue to independent hearing. These devices allow you to break free of your dependence on others, and can make all the difference in strengthening your relationship with those around you rather than fueling unrewarding emotions.

Rejection

Bill was a likeable but boisterous man. He told funny jokes but he told them with such volume that strangers thirty feet away laughed. He was a source of constant entertainment as well as embarrassment to his wife and friends. Sitting in a restaurant, he'd talk about people's personal problems. It wasn't that his friends didn't want their problems discussed, they just didn't want the entire restaurant to hear about it. It was as if Bill had no sense of what was appropriate. No one suspected, until I met Bill, his wife and others for lunch one day, that he had a marked loss of hearing. Bill knew it, but he wasn't about to let anyone else in on his secret. His refusal for help cost him the relationships of people who once truly loved and appreciated him. However, his friends simply could no longer tolerate the humiliations that went with the friendship.

Many hard of hearing people are rejected by others who do not recognize their condition. When others remain uninformed about why you may behave or interact the way you do, they're forced to draw wrong conclusions that carry undesirable consequences. You don't have to be vulnerable to social rejection. You have to experience this only a few times to know how painful it is.

Spouses & Significant Others

If you're an average person with hearing loss, you know that your own impatience at times has caused you to be harsher on loved ones than you'd like, or insensitive, unkind or unfair. Once you've realized what you've done, you may feel guilty. You may wish you could have handled the situation differently but you just couldn't control yourself. You may feel like it's a vicious cycle—you expect loved ones to be your ears, and those around you get fed up doing the hearing for you. No one wins.

When I consult with a person experiencing hearing loss, I turn to the spouse or companion and ask for his or her feelings. The common response is, "I'm so tired of repeating myself!" What you might not know is that everyone feels the same. As stated earlier, others can feel resentful that they must do your work.

Only 20 percent of people who suffer from hearing loss seek treatment through hearing aids. This speaks volumes about what spouses endure. It does not only mean louder television, repeating yourself throughout the day, and filling in parts of important conversations, it dangerously raises the level of anxiety in a healthy spouse married to someone with hearing loss. Your spouse will develop her or his own anxiety around your issues, which can start with annoyance and lead to anger, intolerance, a sense of hopelessness, and can even lead to depression. In some cases it ends in divorce. Struggling to communicate under these circumstances can be exhausting.

Many people with untreated hearing loss feel they are not ready for hearing aids. Inspiring you to seek this needed help may be the most challenging task your spouse and family face. Change can only begin with your readiness, but the rewards can dramatically improve lives and transform relationships.

Expectations Versus Actual Performance

If you're a person living in a non-amplified world, you no doubt have expectations about hearing that may not align with your performance. I've known people with hearing loss refuse to get hearing aids, then go into situations expecting to hear. At the end of the evening, I'd point out how much conversation was missed.

People who haven't yet come to terms with their loss of hearing, or who have not fully admitted this to themselves, mistakenly believe that *they hear all they need to hear.* The truth is, *you only hear what your hearing capacity permits.* The illusion to oneself is two-fold: you not only fail to get important information but you don't even know it. The illusion to others is that they believe communication has occurred when in fact it hasn't. Thus, we have multiple altered realties!

Exercise #2

Here's a little exercise that can help you better understand hearing loss. Divide the top of a blank sheet of paper into three sections: on the left, title it "Situations;" in the middle "Expectations;" and on the right, "Actual Performance."

List three to five situations or environments where you expect to hear regardless of whether or not you actually can. Your task is to rate the items under the "Expectations" and "Actual Performance" columns by selecting one of the following ratings:

NEVER - RARELY - SOMETIMES - OFTEN - ALWAYS

After you've completed this, take another piece of paper and list the same situations. Then have your spouse or someone close to you complete how they think your expectations versus actual performance pan out. This makes for good and healthy discussion, and for excellent comparisons. The more truthful you are with yourself, the more you'll gain from these insights.

Interpretation

If you've rated everything in the exercise the same for all situations, either you're an amazingly well adjusted person with hearing loss, or you're kidding yourself. It's unlikely that all hearing situations on your list will be evaluated equally even if you are well adjusted.

So, take a closer look at your list. Bear in mind that people with normal hearing will rate the situations of expectations and performance differently because of their varying listening environments. The difference indicates the magnitude of the problem; the greater the difference, the greater the problem. For many people with loss of hearing, it's typical to have expectations higher than performance levels. As a result, reactions to environmental situations that prove difficult can lead to the emotions we've discussed.

Acceptance and Moving On

Do you want better communication? Do you want to do more to help yourself? Is the quality of *your* life important enough to *you* to make positive changes? Do you care enough about loved ones to make these changes?

Acceptance of hearing loss allows you to move on. It's that easy. You already recognize the trials and tribulations of insufficient hearing. You know that despite all efforts to compensate for not hearing, nothing gets you through. This realization is essential before you can move on with clear vision. Coming to terms with the emotions surrounding your hearing builds that bridge to healing; and acceptance of your hearing loss allows you safe passage.

References

1. Lilly J. *The Center of the Cyclone: An Autobiography of Inner Space.* New York: Bantam Books, 1972.
2. Kochkin S and Rogin CM. Quantifying the obvious: the impact of hearing instruments on quality of life. The Hearing Review 7(1), 2000.
3. Silman S, et al. Late on-set auditory deprivation: effects of monaural versus binaural hearing aids. J. Acoust. Soc. Am. 76:1357-62, 1984.
4. Silman S, et al. Adult-onset auditory deprivation. J. Am. Acad. Audiol. 3:390-96, 1992.
5. Carmen R and Uram S. Hearing loss and anxiety in adults. The Hearing Journal 55(4), 2002.
6. Reiger DA, Narrow WE, Rae DS, et al. The de facto mental and addictive disorders service system. Epidemiologic Catchment Area prospective 1-year prevalence rates of disorders and services. Archives of General Psychiatry 50(2):85-94.,1993.
7. Klerman GL, Weissman MM. Increasing rates of depression. JAMA 261(15):2229-35, 1989.
8. Bridges JA, Bentler RA. Relating hearing aid use to well-being among older adults. The Hearing Journal 51(7):39-44, 1998.
9. Kochkin S. MarkeTrak VI: The VA and Direct Mail Sales Spark Growth in Hearing Aid Market. The Hearing Review 8(12), 2001.

CHAPTER TWO

How to Obtain Professional Help
Robert E. Sandlin, Ph.D.

Dr. Sandlin received his Ph.D. in Clinical Audiology from Wayne State University in 1961. He serves as an Adjunct Professor of Audiology at San Diego State University. He has served as a research and clinical audiologist in several clinics and hospitals. He served as Director of the California Tinnitus Assessment in San Diego that is devoted to developing effective strategies for the non-medical management of those with subjective tinnitus. Dr. Sandlin has published over 90 articles and edited four major texts on hearing aid sciences and amplification, and contributed a number of chapters to other texts His greatest achievement has been six tremendous children and seven grandchildren who provide a constant source of satisfaction for him and his wife, Joann.

In the first edition of this book, I suggested procedures and reasons for finding the most qualified individual to help you along the way. You may ask, "Are there more things that I can do to help me find the best person who understands my hearing problems?"

Yes!

There are things you may want to consider in your search for professional guidance. This is especially true, in view of the improvements in hearing aid design and function. What I mean is that advances in hearing aid technology may be very helpful to those with hearing loss.

Why is this so important to you? Hearing aids with computer capability are now available that permit the hearing professional to help you in ways that were impossible before. The fancy name for this advanced hearing aid is *Digital Signal Processing*.

The task of finding the most qualified individual to manage whatever hearing problems you have is not as difficult as it might first seem. Your biggest challenge will be narrowing your search down from a lot of choices to a few options. In doing so, you'll reduce your frustrations and sharpen your focus on what's required. There is always a certain amount of frustration in seeking help for some human ailment. Questions may arise for which there are no immediate answers. For example, have you ever asked yourself any of the following questions?

- Do I need a hearing aid at all?
- Do I need two?
- How do I know if the recommended hearing aids are the best for me?
- How do I know whether the person I'm going to see is competent?
- How do I determine if the person I'm seeing really cares about me or is merely profit-motivated?
- What if I don't like the hearing aids, what action can I take?
- How can I determine whether medicine or surgery can improve my hearing?

These questions are not uncommon. The important thing is that all of them can be answered in an intelligent manner. A lot depends on whom you select to be your personal hearing healthcare manager. Your physician can tell if medicine or surgery would help. The audiologist can verify the presence or absence of a significant hearing loss and select and dispense the appropriate hearing aid. The hearing instrument specialist is also qualified to select, fit and dispense hearing aids.

Be optimistic about your potential success with hearing aids. Think of all the benefits you could experience. Look at it this way. You've already won more than half the battle just by making a positive decision to do something.

The purpose of this chapter is to suggest ways in which you can connect to the proper hearing care professionals, and understand what they can offer. This will require positive action on your part, defined as taking a step(s) to successfully eliminate or reduce your hearing problem.

This chapter will provide guidance to you and your family on several key issues. In the process, it should reduce your fears, apprehensions and frustrations sometimes associated with any search for better ways to manage a health problem. By the end of this chapter, you should be knowledgeable about how to move through the maze of hearing healthcare professionals. You should know who's who in this profession. You should be able to establish who is the best person to meet your particular needs. You will know how to determine the qualifications of the provider who might best serve you.

If you have doubts or problems regarding the hearing healthcare person you elected to see, get a second opinion. You know your hearing is extremely important to you. You have every right to find the best help possible. Not all hearing health professionals have the same amount of knowledge and experience. Let's review some history underlying the emergence of hearing aid dispensing as an occupation in the United States.

History of Hearing Aid Dispensing

The selection and fitting of hearing aids has been practiced for well over seventy years. During that period of time, there have been steady improvements in the design and performance of hearing aid devices. However, less than twenty-five years ago, hearing aid dispensers were not required to have any special technical training to carry out the necessary tasks for selection and fitting of hearing aids. Nor was it required for the individual to have a dedicated place of business. Only sufficient capital to buy hearing aids from a manufacturer and go into business were needed. Further, early on, there was no sophisticated diagnostic or hearing aid measuring equipment required to validate the degree of improvement provided by hearing aids or to qualify their acoustic performance.

As the manufacturing of hearing instruments became more technologically advanced, so did the ability to measure their electroacoustic characteristics. As time passed, manufacturers initiated training programs in the proper selection and fitting of their hearing aid products. For the most part, early educational programs provided by the industry were very instrumental in improving selection and fitting skills. The manufacturer was interested, primarily, in it's own product and most educational efforts were dictated by that philosophy.

Nevertheless, from the early introduction of hearing aids and the early selection and fitting practices, those who had less than positive experiences regarding hearing aid use developed some negative attitudes. While some of these attitudes may have had a basis in fact, it's important for you to know that significant and positive changes have come about within the hearing aid dispensing field. For example, by the late 1970s, most individuals who dispensed hearing instruments were licensed by the state in which they practiced. In order to receive a hearing aid dispensing license, a test of basic competency had to be passed.

Today, these tests have become more sophisticated. Area of study includes a basic understanding of the anatomy, physiology, neurology pathology of the hearing system. They also include factors contributing to hearing impairment; psychology of the hearing-impaired person; and electroacoustic measurement of hearing aid devices.

In addition, other areas of study include administering and understanding hearing tests; understanding audiometric test results for the purpose of fitting hearing aids; learning effective counseling strategies; and becoming familiar with state laws governing the professional activities of hearing instrument providers. These tests are not exhaustive ones nor necessarily overly difficult but did cover basic educational requirements. Licensure to fit hearing aids created a higher level of competence.

There are two individual and distinct disciplines now dispensing hearing aids: the Clinical Audiologist and the Hearing Instrument Specialist (HIS). Let's look at both of these practitioners.

Hearing Instrument Specialists

There are thousands of qualified hearing instrument specialists throughout the United States. State requirements and licensing assures that they are knowledgeable and capable of performing necessary measurements for the selection and fitting of hearing aids. Many are members of the International Hearing Society (IHS). In order to qualify and maintain membership in this group, continuing education is mandatory. The hearing instrument specialist also can pursue additional training to achieve Board Certification (BC) status. In order for members to be board certified, a written examination must be taken and passed. This examination is more demanding of specific knowledge than is the examination of individual states.

It can be stated positively that the hearing instrument specialist is much more qualified to select and fit these devices than they were at any time in the past. This qualification has been largely based on state licensure and mandatory continuing education requirements. Much of the credit is due to the continuing efforts of the International Hearing Society and its board certification program. Additionally, state certification has advanced the professional status of the hearing aid specialist and has inspired greater consumer confidence.

History of Audiology

Although the medical profession has long been interested in the measurement of hearing loss for the purpose of diagnosis and treatment, there was no great effort until World War II to establish a separate branch of medicine dealing solely with the objective assessment of the human auditory system. At that time, hundreds, if not thousands of returning servicemen had incurred permanent hearing impairment due to the injuries of war.

Physicians recognized the value of assessing hearing because of its implications regarding medical management. It soon became evident that most hearing loss caused by battle conditions could not be treated medically or surgically. This was so because most of the injuries to the ear were caused by shell blasts and other loud, explosive noises. As an aside, do you know that once nerve cells in the ear die, they cannot be replaced? I mention this because the majority of people with hearing impairment have received damage to the ear, which causes some of the nerve cells to die.

Because of the number of servicemen and women with hearing loss, there needed to be some organized, clinical program. A program was needed which could evaluate the type and degree of hearing loss as well as develop effective rehabilitation programs. Just the sheer numbers of servicemen needing immediate attention gave need to program development. Advanced techniques of measuring hearing loss were introduced. More sophisticated equipment was developed for the measurement of hearing. Much attention was given to rehabilitation programs which would permit, as much as possible, the hard of hearing serviceman to live effectively in a hearing world. You can imagine the important role that hearing aids played in the successful rehabilitation of these servicemen and women.

Coupled with the urgency to meet the needs of the hard of hearing soldier was the need to provide expanded training for personnel working in rehabilitation programs for hearing-impaired veterans. As training programs were established and proved to be very worthwhile, a name—a professional label—had to be associated with those who performed these services. A branch of special education merged with medicine and this new academic discipline emerged as the profession of Audiology.

Since those early beginnings, the practice of audiology has expanded tremendously. The amount of audiological research is reflected in the number of scientific journals devoted solely to its study. The growth of this field is evident by the significant increase in academic programs in hearing science.

It's noteworthy that audiologists have been responsible for almost all of the formal research efforts involving hearing aid use and function. Yet, they were prevented from dispensing hearing aids for profit by their national association, the American Speech-Language-Hearing Association (ASHA).

But all businesses, whether medical or not, are profit driven, and rightfully so or they could no longer afford to keep their doors open. In the early 1970s, many audiologists recognized this. Whether it was naive of the ASHA or an outdated ideology, the time had come for hearing aids to be part of clinical audiology practice. Several clinical audiologists in the United States opposed the majority viewpoint and began to dispense hearing aids. They believed they had the right to include dispensing in their responsibilities to consumers. Those audiologists who dispensed hearing aids had their clinical certification revoked by ASHA.

However, by 1978, as more and more audiologists had adopted the dispensing philosophy, ASHA revised their Code of Ethics and accepted hearing aids as being an integral part of the services offered by audiologists. Since that time, audiology has had an enormous and positive influence on the hearing aid industry. Hearing aid evaluation and subsequent dispensing of hearing aids are now considered to be well within the scope of practice for audiologists.

Clinical Audiologists

Audiologists are familiar with the functions of the human auditory system and trained to understand normal and abnormal functions of that system. They are trained to perform routine and, at times, highly technical diagnostic tests to determine what is causing abnormal auditory function. Their depth of understanding of the physiology, neurology, anatomy and pathology of the auditory system is greater than that of the hearing instrument specialist. This is true because of the required education.

Further, audiologists provide rehabilitation to those with hearing loss ranging in degrees from mild to profound. Over the past 15 to 20 years, the field of audiology has expanded to include the assessment of hearing loss for the purpose of selecting and fitting hearing aid devices.

The advanced training and educational requirements are

dictated by ASHA. To obtain a Master's Degree in Audiology, typically six years of study at an approved university or college are required. In addition, the student must serve a clinical fellowship year and must pass a rigorous examination. Audiologists must earn at least a Master's Degree to assume clinical or academic responsibilities.

Also, several universities offer a Doctor of Philosophy (Ph.D.) degree as the terminal degree requiring two to four years of additional study. However, in the mid-1990s, there was a concerted effort by a group of audiologists to establish one common professional degree by which all "clinical" audiologists would be recognized—the Doctor of Audiology (Au.D.). The consensus is that by around 2012, the primary degree to be granted by most audiology programs will in fact be the Au.D. The Ph.D. will then be a direction for those audiologists wishing to pursue teaching and research.

Academic preparation stresses the diagnostic procedures required to differentiate various pathologies of the auditory system. This may include anything from wax in the ear canal to a tumor resting on the eighth cranial nerve. For most academic programs, audiology also includes rehabilitation programs for the deaf and hard of hearing.

More recently, academic programs relating to the electroacoustic performance, selection, assessment and fitting of hearing aids have been added to the curriculum. Inclusion of hearing aid dispensing as an integral part of audiology practice began in the early 1980s and has continued to grow in acceptance.

Similarities Among Providers

In those states requiring licensure, both the audiologist and hearing instrument specialist must pass the same mandatory examination and complete the required number of continuing education hours each year to maintain licensure. Members of both groups must abide by the same standards of ethical practice and are subject to the same state laws governing the dispensing of hearing aids. (Did you know that in states where licensing is mandatory, the physician must also be licensed to dispense hearing aids?)

One significant similarity is that each group has access to the same hearing instrument manufacturers and to all literature and clinical information pertaining to hearing aids and their electroacoustic performance. There are no restrictions placed on which manufacturer can provide hearing aid devices to those who dispense.

There are, however, a few manufacturers of hearing instruments who will sell their product only to approved franchises. The basic philosophy underlying a given franchise operation is that it's more efficient for the manufacturer to deal with persons dispensing only their product.

Obviously, there are pros and cons to this argument, but very active franchises do exist in today's marketplace. All practitioners have access to pertinent scientific and trade journals and may very well modify that which they do in the selection and fitting process based on information contained in specific articles. Most hearing instrument dispensers and dispensing audiologists have more than a single brand of hearing aids available to their clients.

From a humanistic point of view, I think you will find that each discipline is sensitive to your needs. Each individual will do his or her best to satisfy your needs and maintain your confidence in their abilities.

A Difference Among Providers

The major difference as already alluded to, is that of formal education. The hearing instrument specialist does not have a formal educational background in measuring the performance of the human auditory system for purposes of diagnosis or in the rehabilitation of those with hearing impairment. He or she is more typically required to have a high school education in order to sit for the examination to qualify as a dispenser. This description of the academic requirements of a hearing instrument specialist is not intended as an indictment of the qualifications necessary to become a provider, nor is it intended as a yardstick against which to measure proficiency in the selection and fitting of hearing aid devices. Rather, it's a straightforward statement of criteria imposed by most states in granting licensure to those qualifying by examination to dispense hearing aids. There are thousands of qualified hearing instrument specialists throughout the United States. By far, the majority is knowledgeable and capable of performing necessary measurements to select the most appropriate hearing instruments.

The education required to become a clinical audiologist is extensive. It entails undergraduate and graduate school training in assessing neurophysiologic function and dysfunction of the hearing system through the administration of defined clinical tests. Audiology is, and has been for decades, a recognized academic discipline.

Inherent in the training of audiologists is courses relating to hearing aid amplification. A number of training institutions provide clinical practicum for their graduate students in hearing instrument dispensing and specific courses relating to selection and fitting of amplification devices.

It's gratifying to report to you that many more major universities are offering academic courses dealing with the selection, measurement and dispensing of hearing aids. Hearing instrument dispensing is now well within the scope of audiologic practice.

Your Significant Other

When starting your search for qualified service providers, it may be wise to consider taking another person with you. It can be your spouse or another family member or friend. This person can be a second pair of eyes and ears to assist in the evaluation process. He or she may be able to provide a somewhat more objective observation of the hearing care provider's skills and services. This person can serve as a sounding board to respond to such questions as, "What do you think I should do?" or "Should I get one or two hearing aids?"

Finding The Preferred Professional

In the selection of a qualified provider, you want someone who demonstrates proficiency and competence. You must realize that you'll be using hearing aid amplification for many years to come, and therefore, will want to establish a long-term relationship with whomever you choose. This is something to which you should give considerable thought.

Listed below are some of the recommended criteria you can use to select the best person in whom you can place confidence and trust. These are the essential components that you should look for when seeking a hearing care professional:

Expectations of Your Hearing Care Provider

Hearing aid researchers agree that the interaction of the hearing aid fitter and the client is a critical element in successful hearing aid use. There are specific elements to this important relationship that are common to providers who achieve a high degree of satisfaction among their clients. Successful providers believe in the efficacy (benefit) of hearing aids and they keep up with rapid changes in hearing aid technology.

Expect your hearing health provider to have an attractive and clean office with convenient business hours. Expect him or her to act professionally, to be knowledgeable and demonstrate the benefits I will present in the next section.

Expect your provider to be able to explain hearing aid options to you in simple terms. Demonstrations are often helpful which allow you to listen to a particular type of circuitry, to compare different settings in noise, or to experience the difference between monaural (one hearing aid) and binaural amplification. A good professional dispensing hearing aids never assumes that clients cannot understand complex concepts. You should be given as much information as you require in the form of discussion, videotapes, books, brochures, consumer guides, and technical articles. Currently, there's a popular phrase, "too much information." There's also a time to stop giving information. Not all patients want or need a bus load of materials. Information needs to be tailored to your needs.

Research has identified that stigma is still a very common reason why people hold back from purchasing hearing aids. It's very important that you're allowed to express your feelings about how hearing aids will look and what you think about them. Simply talking about your feelings associated with your hearing loss can be of tremendous benefit. Some people don't care what size or style of hearing aid is chosen. Others are extremely conscious about the cosmetic aspect. (Sociologist Dr. Cuzzort in Chapter 8 offers valuable insights on stigma.)

Experienced providers know how to motivate skeptical, timid hearing aid candidates. They know that proactive clients have a higher likelihood of becoming satisfied hearing aid wearers. All providers want their clients to be willing to go the distance, even if they make a few mistakes in the beginning. Sometimes the process can be difficult. A caring professional will always see you through, if you will.

Optimizing the match between your lifestyle and communication needs is an important determination by your provider, something which can have direct impact on you. We're all more likely to trust someone who we feel understands us. Therefore, effective hearing care providers are good listeners. It's important that your provider takes the time to learn what problems you have in meetings, groups, theater, with co-workers, family, and in your place of worship.

It's also important for you to express what you hope to improve in your hearing world as a result of amplification.

Once you have been fit with hearing aids, it is absolutely mandatory that the person who fit you with the hearing aids explain in detail how to care for the hearing aid, how to clean and maintain them, how to use the switches or remote (if there is one), and how to change batteries. You should receive an instructional booklet for later referral after the initial counseling or instructional session.

Especially with programmable hearing aids, it's not uncommon to come back several times in order to get "just the right fit" (physical, acoustical, audiological) for you. This is a normal part of the hearing aid fitting process. Multiple adjustments to hearing aids are normal and are not indicative of a "lemon." However, it's important that these adjustments occur during the normal trial period, and that you are satisfied the product meets your needs.

Years of Service

If somebody has been providing hearing services for many years, it generally is an indicator that many people with hearing loss have been seen by that person. Although it may not necessarily indicate superior knowledge and care, it does suggest that this person has been in business awhile and is not likely to disappear tomorrow. As with any skill-related work, the longer you do it, the more proficient you become.

In the selection process, you may want to determine the years of service a particular practitioner has in providing amplification devices to those with hearing loss. However, I must tell you that years of service does not always mean that the person is the most qualified to work with, or the one who understands the latest in technological advances in hearing aid performance. Don't hesitate to ask anyone from whom you are seeking advice and direction to review his or her professional and academic background.

Level of Knowledge

It's in your best interest to determine the level of skill one has in the selection and fitting of hearing aids. Just having a state license to dispense hearing instruments does not guarantee that the individual is current with technological advances in hearing aid performance. In the past decade or so, there have been significant changes in this industry. You should not feel uncomfortable, and the provider should not feel challenged, if you inquire about his or her level of knowledge as it pertains to current hearing aid selection and use.

As a matter of fact, many hearing instrument providers may display a variety of certificates indicating they've taken specific courses of study to become more competent. You should take advantage of this by carefully noting the dates on these certificates. A certificate hanging on the wall may not tell you how much the person learned, but it does indicate that he or she continues to study. If you observe that there is nothing to indicate continuing education, simply ask what his or her continuing education has been.

Empathy and Compassion

Your hearing aid needs are best met by an empathetic person who understands what you are experiencing. There is really no substitute for empathy. If the hearing health professional is truly empathetic to your needs, he or she will do what is necessary to achieve the greatest benefit to you.

Although similar in meaning, compassion is a deep sympathetic concern or feeling for a given condition or for an individual, while empathy is more of an intellectual acceptance and understanding of an individual's need or given condition. In essence, you want services rendered by someone who really understands how you feel.

Temperament and Likeability

For our purposes, temperament can be defined as the natural and predictable behavior of an individual. As it relates to one's needs when searching for answers to hearing loss problem, it is the overt actions of the individual. By this I mean that the hearing health professional should display patience, understanding and concern, without eliciting fear or unrealistic statements regarding hearing aid use.

Certainly, knowledge of hearing aid dispensing is fundamental to doing business and meeting hearing aid needs. But a very important and essential ingredient is also the temperament and likeability of the one with whom you are doing business. Likeability is a sense of joy or contentment in the presence of an individual who expresses a sincere interest in your needs and feelings. It is not something that can always be expressed in concrete terms. It's something you feel and experience in a very positive way.

The sense of feeling positive about the hearing healthcare professional cannot be regulated by a state agency. Like a physician with good bedside manners, you want professionals who conduct themselves in a way that allows you to feel protected. You want this person to be sensitive to your needs. You want to feel comfortable revealing your very private feelings regarding hearing aid use. You don't want to feel like you're intruding, but rather, that the hearing health professional appreciates the opportunity to serve you. It's in your best interest to gather a good sense about the person with whom you are expected to work closely.

Dependability

Although seldom discussed in hearing aid literature, dependability is a very important attribute to successful patient management. That is, as a patient, can you depend on your hearing healthcare professional to be there when you need him or her? Does their office have predictable hours? Is the dispenser there every day of the week or just on certain days? Does the dispenser provide emergency care just in case something goes wrong with the hearing aid? You may consider talking to others who have purchased hearing aids from the dispenser and question them about dependability.

The large majority of dispensers are dependable. They are interested in providing services when you need them and want you to feel free to call them when a need arises. To the dispenser, it is simply good business practice to maintain a high level of dependability.

Talk to Successful Users

It was stated earlier in this chapter that all hearing losses are not the same. Regardless of the degree and type of hearing loss you may have, others with permanent hearing loss can tell you of their experiences with a given practitioner and whether or not they were satisfied with the services offered and the benefits received. Ask people who have utilized hearing aids for several years. They have experienced the contributions and limitations of technological advances in hearing aid design and performance. They can be a rich resource for you.

Be careful though, because the positive experience of one person does not mean you will have a positive experience with the same hearing aid or the same professional. Conversely, the negative report by a friend doesn't preclude you will also have a bad experience. The emotional and physical needs for all with hearing loss are not the same. You may differ a great deal in your emotional reactions, as well as your acceptance and use of hearing aids.

Make it a point to talk to your friends and others who use hearing aids. Not only can these folks be supportive of your pursuit and use of amplification but you may learn from their positive, real life experiences how best to adjust to and benefit from hearing aid amplification. You may also learn a great deal from their mistakes.

Background Check

As would be true in any profession, if you're uncertain about the audiologist, hearing instrument specialist or the physician providing services to you, contact the Better Business Bureau in your community or directly contact the state committee responsible for hearing aid licensure. You may also check with the International Hearing Society (HIS), American Speech-Language-Hearing Association (ASHA) or the American Academy of Audiology. (These institutions and more are listed in Appendix II.)

Further, in many states, hearing instrument specialists and audiologists have their own Ethics Committee. By contacting this committee, you can find out if complaints have been registered against a given provider and how such complaints were resolved.

Spur of the Moment Decisions

At times, some people proceed with a hearing aid evaluation and the subsequent purchase of hearing aids on a spur of the moment decision. Such a spontaneous reaction in some people is exactly what is required to get the task done. But much will depend on your own temperament. If you're a person who doesn't like to spend a lot of time mulling things over, and you know what you need, such an impulsive decision to take quick action may work well for you.

On the other hand, you may need more time to think about a plan of action. Some people may have to muster the courage (or even the finances) to do something about their problem. That's okay. A few extra days of deciding what course to follow or how to arrange it won't make any difference. No doubt it has taken you years to get to this point anyway. You will find the professional person who will meet all qualifications you need and demand.

Yellow Pages

Some consumers consult the yellow pages and select the individual whose advertisement is most visually attractive or largest or the individual who seems to have the best credentials. Others may select the first business beginning with "A." The value of yellow pages is for you to ascertain "who's who" in your community. Examine your options and proceed with optimism and faith in yourself that you have discerned the best choice.

Medical Practitioners

Many people prefer to begin their hearing healthcare journey with the family physician whom they've known for years and who's judgment they trust. This seems like an intelligent decision because you would believe that your family physician would refer you to a hearing aid provider if needed.

However, as Dr. Carmen previously pointed out, many physicians do not refer their patients to hearing healthcare practitioners for the purpose of obtaining hearing aids. Most of these well-meaning physicians *falsely* believe you cannot be helped. If this has been your experience, I would suggest you seek a second opinion (from an audiologist or hearing instrument specialist). Some physicians are not current with state-of-the-art technology regarding hearing aids, and fail to recognize the benefit they provide to hard of hearing persons.

Nevertheless, if something about your ears or hearing is in need of specific medical attention, you could be referred to a medical specialist whose primary concern is the diagnosis and treatment of impaired hearing and diseases of the ear. Such a specialist is an otologist. The otologist restricts his or her practice to problems associated with the auditory system. The otolaryngologist is also a specialist in treating diseases of the ear, but treats nose and throat disorders as well. While either can provide you with adequate treatment, otologists are even more specialized in their training.

If your physician or medical specialist refers you to someone for hearing aids, it should be safely assumed that the practitioner knows you will receive competent care. If you have any doubts about such a referral, you should ask your physician whatever questions are on your mind.

The Medical Waiver

If you're an experienced hearing aid wearer and you're being issued new hearing aids, federal law does not mandate that a physician see you. This is because the government takes for granted that by now you're experienced enough to recognize the presence of a problem, which needs medical attention. New users may not be as knowledgeable. In light of potential problems, federal law requires that anyone dispensing hearing aids be able to recognize a number of fairly obvious conditions of the ears. (See Chapter 8 Question & Answers number 7 for further information.) If a medical condition is recognized by your provider, you can be assured that you'll be referred for treatment prior to issuance of hearing aids.

If you're a first-time hearing aid wearer, federal law allows you to visit a hearing aid provider without first being seen by a physician, so long as you sign a waiver of medical evaluation for hearing. This essentially states, "You are being advised that the Food and Drug Administration has determined that your best health interests would be served if you had a medical evaluation by a licensed physician prior to purchasing hearing aids."

The waiver serves two solid purposes. First, it alerts you, the consumer, to the fact that a potentially serious medical problem could exist, and should not be overlooked, especially if you have any ear symptoms. Second, if you were recently seen in a physician's office and you know there's nothing wrong with your ears (other than hearing loss), you shouldn't have to go back through the medical route to obtain approval for a hearing aid purchase. Many consumers feel that a medical visit under these circumstances is both unnecessary, even redundant, and simply adds to the cost. By signing the waiver, you exercise the right to make your own decision.

A Hearing Evaluation

There are a number of hearing tests that an audiologist or hearing instrument specialist can do to determine how severe you're hearing loss is. Please keep in mind that all tests administered are necessary in order to make the most appropriate assessment of your hearing and find the best approach to meet your hearing aid needs. In essentially all cases, you should have no pain or discomfort during the administration of diagnostic tests.

Please note that all tests performed are for the purpose of selecting and fitting hearing aids. The primary purpose of a hearing aid evaluation is simply that of determining whether you're a reasonable candidate for hearing aid use. Another purpose is that of determining the type of hearing aid most appropriate to your needs.

Otoscopic Examination

Prior to the administration of hearing tests, your hearing healthcare provider should perform a routine otoscopic examination. Its purpose is to visually examine the status of your ear. It takes only a few minutes to complete and adds a great deal of understanding to what may have caused your hearing loss. The otoscope is a hand-held instrument about the size of a standard flashlight. Some are connected to a large-screen monitor like a TV, enabling you to see as well. It casts a sharply focused light into the ear that illuminates the canal and reveals its condition.

Some otoscopes have greater magnification and provide the examiner with a more precise view of anatomical structures. Such views may suggest problems that need to be attended to. For example, a build-up of earwax may be viewed blocking sound from entering the ear. Naturally, the greater the skill and training of the professional performing the otoscopy, the greater the chances are that existing problems will be identified.

Another major contribution of an otoscopic examination is that of assessing the status of the eardrum. For example, there could be a hole (perforation) in the eardrum due to some traumatic incident or disease process. The size and location of the hole can affect one's ability to hear well enough to understand all that is being said. Further, otoscopic examination can detect the presence of fluid in the middle ear space. Middle ear fluids can greatly reduce your ability to hear sounds at a normal level. Unfortunately, middle ear fluids can become diseased through bacterial invasion and cause serious medical problems.

Please keep in mind that an otoscopic inspection by an audiologist or hearing instrument specialist is not a diagnostic procedure. Only a qualified physician can do that. But if the hearing health professional sees something suggesting a medical condition, he or she must refer you to a physician.

Listening for Tones

Following otoscopic examination, a number of specialized hearing tests may be conducted. The purpose of hearing tests is to determine how much hearing loss you have, if any, and what is the probable cause. Usually, the basic hearing test consists of sitting in a sound-treated chamber, listening to a series of tones, and indicating to the professional when you've heard them. Some tones will be low frequency (low pitch) and others will be high (high pitch). As you know by now, if you have a hearing loss, you won't be able to hear all of the tones at normal intensity levels. Also, you will not know how well or poorly you've done until the test is completed.

The lowest tones that the human ear can detect are very close to the sensation of feeling. At the other end of the continuum, a young healthy person can hear tones even higher than the highest violin note. We don't actually need to hear at either of these two extremes, but we do need hearing intact in the middle range where speech sounds vibrate.

Most people have greater difficulty hearing high frequencies. This is readily demonstrated by listening to (without looking at) someone repeat vowel sounds which are all low frequency, such as /a/, /e/, /i/, /o/ and /u/. Now have them produce the utterance of higher frequency sounds which make up consonants like /sh/, /ch/ and /s/ for example. Sixty-five percent of audible speech intelligibility comes from consonant (high frequency) sounds. Putting all of this in context, have someone repeat the words /sheath/, /cheap/ and /sheet/. If you can't hear the very subtle differences between these words, you will readily appreciate and recognize how important every sound is in adding information to what you hear. You might now also suspect a high frequency loss.

Listening for Speech

As you well know, there's a direct correlation between the level of your hearing loss and your ability to understand words when presented at normal speech levels. Therefore, a couple of tests will be performed to assess your ability to understand selected words. The Speech Reception Threshold (SRT) test entails repeating two-syllable words such as "hotdog," "baseball," or "downtown."

On this particular test, the more familiar you are with the words, the more accurate the results (you just won't be able to predict which order the words will come). These words are presented at progressively weaker volume levels until you're forced to guess at what you think the words are. The value of this test is to determine how soft certain words can be made before you can only repeat them correctly 50 percent of the time. This point is called threshold. It's used as a working reference for the amount of power that eventually will be needed in your hearing aids, and can allow a certain degree of predictable success you may have in their use.

Another test is the Word Discrimination Score (WDS). Fifty one-syllable words such as "wet," "chew," or "car," are presented for you to repeat. The lower your score, the greater your difficulty in hearing and understanding people who talk with you. Usually a score poorer than 88 percent would indicate that you have at least some difficulty in some situations. None of the words on this test will be repeated if you miss them. The number of words repeated correctly reflects how well you understand speech under ideal listening conditions. Word discrimination tests are basic to good clinical practice. These tests tell us what your ability is to understand speech without hearing aids. Once you are fit with hearing aids, the same word discrimination test will tell us how much improvement occurs.

Assessment of Middle Ear Structures

In a complete diagnostic evaluation of your hearing, other tests may be carried out to determine how well your hearing system is performing. Typically, clinical audiologists conduct these tests on highly sophisticated equipment. In certain cases, it may be important for your practitioner to know if the eardrum is moving appropriately when sounds strike it. If some disease or pathology affects the way in which the eardrum (or other structures) move, then we want to be able to identify and measure it.

Special diagnostic equipment is used through which primarily two objectives are accomplished: mobility of the eardrum (assessed by increasing air pressure into the outer ear canal), and integrity of the inner ear (by means of a series of loud tones to try to trigger your acoustic reflex). Both the pressure tests and presence or absence of the acoustic reflex add information to the final diagnosis of your hearing problem.

If these basic hearing tests confirm a loss of hearing or abnormal function, then further testing, including x-rays, blood samples, or certain brain function tests may be conducted to gain even more specific information about your hearing problem and what may be done about it. The purpose of these various tests is to compare your results with those of normal hearing persons. By making this comparison, your practitioner can quickly determine if you have normal hearing or some degree of loss.

Since you might have already suspected a hearing problem anyway, these tests will confirm your suspicions. Even though some people are apprehensive in general about taking tests, let me assure you that these diagnostic procedures recommended by your audiologist or otologist can be critical in arriving at a competent diagnosis of your problem and its proper management. In most cases, sophisticated tests are not needed to determine your hearing status or the type of hearing aids best suited to meet your needs.

So, don't be overwhelmed by all these tests. They are a necessary part of your quest for better hearing.

Medical and/or Surgical Treatment

In many cases, hearing tests along with other information your practitioner has gathered may indicate the need for medical or surgical management. For the most part, this is good news, for it means that such intervention could resolve your problem and restore your hearing to a normal or near-normal state. If such is the case, there is usually no need for hearing aids. However, let's assume you have seen the otologist and are told that nothing medically or surgically can be done to treat your hearing problem. What can you now do to improve your ability to hear and understand? In the final analysis, when a hearing loss exists that cannot be successfully treated by medicine or surgery, the use of hearing aid amplification is the recommended path to follow.

Conclusions

I have discussed many things you may experience in your search for professional care. It can be a highly rewarding journey if you initiate the process of help. The first step in receiving help is looking for it. And little help can be offered if you fail to deal honestly with the problem. Be assured that you'll be rewarded in your willingness to use amplification by significantly improving your ability to understand much more of your acoustic world. Your frequent requests to have conversations repeated should be markedly fewer, and your blueprint to secure a bridge to healing can at last be fulfilled.

CHAPTER THREE
Mapping Your Own Audiogram
Kris English, Ph.D.

Dr. English earned her Doctorate in Education in 1993 from San Diego State University at Claremont Graduate University. She is an assistant professor at the University of Pittsburgh, and also teaches a class on the Internet for Central Michigan University/Vanderbilt University Bill Wilkerson Center. She has authored four books, three chapters, and over 40 papers, most lately addressing the adjustment process to living with hearing loss. She is currently developing a counseling tool to help children with hearing loss talk to audiologists about hearing aid use, friendships, and self-concept. She and her husband live in constant amazement that their two children are now adults and managing life on their own just fine.

Understanding how to read your own audiogram will assist you in better understanding your personal hearing challenges. At first, this might seem complicated, but it really is quite easy and straightforward. In my discussion with you, I will present "Mini-Summaries" of each section, provided throughout to review vocabulary and concepts, and occasionally "Audiogram Alerts" are provided to highlight a particular point of concern. In time, you will be an expert in describing your audiogram. So let's work together in this exploration.

An audiogram has three main components:
1. A range of pitches, from low to high.
2. A measurement of loudness, from soft to very loud.
3. Your hearing levels for each pitch for each ear.

Audiogram Components
Audiogram Component #1: Pitch
The first component of the audiogram is the range of pitches presented in the hearing test. Wearing headphones (or maybe insert earphones), you heard a series of beeps that may have reminded you of notes on a piano. Some had very low pitches (like the deep bass notes on the left end of the piano keys), some were very high pitches (similar to the far right end of piano keys), and some were in between. These pitches are lined up on the horizontal part of the audiogram, as shown in Figure 3-1.

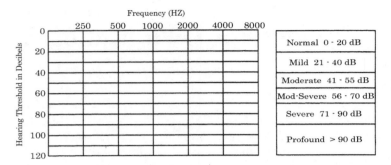

Figure 3-1: Pitch and loudness on an audiogram.

Another term used to describe these beeps is "pure tones." You may have noticed each beep was like a single note on a piano, with no chords or harmonics. The human ear can hear pure tones much lower and higher than the ones shown on the audiogram, but it would take too much time to test them all. For efficiency's sake we focus on what people are most interested in hearing—human speech. So the pure tones found in human speech are selected for testing and are the ones reported on your audiogram.

It may seem a little strange to say these pure tones have anything to do with human speech, but when analyzed electronically, each speech sound has been found to be a unique and complex combination of these pure tones. That's why your hearing care professional started with pure tone testing, as a way to describe the "building blocks" of your hearing ability.

Chances are, the term "frequency" was used during an explanation of your hearing test. For example, you may have been told you have a "high frequency hearing loss." Frequency means pitch: a way of expressing the number of cycles per second (cps) a sound wave occurs in one second. A sound that vibrates your eardrum at 500 times per second (cps) is perceived by our brain as having a low pitch, like the hum of the motor in your refrigerator. As the vibrations per second increase, the pitch of the sound will seem higher and higher, like the cheep of a bird.

A scientist named Heinrich Hertz (1857-1894) described this idea of low and high pitches having different cycles per second, and in his honor, his initials are now used to replace *cps* with *Hz*. So, for example, your hearing test may indicate that you have a hearing loss at 8000 Hz. Because this pitch (frequency) occurs in the higher end of the area for speech sounds, it can also be said to be a high frequency hearing loss.

Mini-Summary

All of these terms mean the same thing:
- A high frequency hearing loss
- A hearing loss in the higher pitches
- A hearing loss at 4000-8000 Hz

Audiogram Component #2: Loudness

The first question we want to answer is: how loud does each pitch have to be for you to hear it? Loudness is recorded on the vertical part of the audiogram (See: Figure 3-1). The unit of measure for loudness is the decibel (abbreviated dB). The audiogram uses increments of 5 dB mainly because the human ear is not usually able to notice differences of less than 5 dB.

This vertical measurement often causes some confusion. The softest levels of hearing are at the top, so the loudness *increases* as it goes *down* the scale. Initially, it might seem more logical to place the softest levels on the bottom and then, as loudness goes up, the scale should go up. So watch for this, and remember: when the loudness of the pitch needs to be increased, it means the hearing level is dropping downward.

Mini-Summary

- Pitch or frequency is measured in Hertz (Hz).
- Loudness is measured in decibels (dB).
- These two measures are combined to tell us how loud (in dB) you need each frequency (Hz) to be in order to just barely hear it. This is called your hearing threshold for that frequency, and will be explained further in the next section.

Audiogram Component #3: Your Hearing in Each Ear

Hearing tests usually start with the middle pitch, 1000 Hz. Let's say your right ear is being tested first. The tester sets the equipment to this frequency, and you raise your finger or push a button every time you hear it. The pure tone gets softer and softer, until you can barely perceive it. That level is your *threshold* for that frequency. Threshold means the softest level you could perceive it.

If your threshold for 1000 Hz is 30 dB, the tester records it with a circle at the intersection of those two values (See: Figure 3-2). Another threshold is then obtained at 2000 Hz, in this example, 40 dB. This procedure is repeated for each frequency. Then the other ear is tested in the same way.

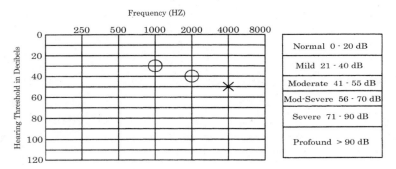

Figure 3-2: Three thresholds.

In Figure 3-2, the "X" found at 45 dB at 4000 Hz represents a threshold for the left ear. How will you remember which symbol is for which ear? The letter *R* will keep things straight: the *right* ear uses a *round* symbol (the circle). And if the hearing care professional used headphones to test your hearing, the *red* headphone went on your *right* ear. It's easy to remember because the "R" is the first letter in **r**ed, **r**ight and **r**ound—*aha!* Once you know the "round" symbols describe the right ear's hearing levels, by default you know the "X" stands for left ear hearing levels.

You may have had your hearing tested not only with headphones or inserts, but also with a bone oscillator that typically rested on your mastoid bone (behind your ear on the skull). The hearing information obtained with the oscillator would be reported with carats "<" and ">" or brackets "[" and "]." They are not included here in our first few audiograms in order to make this a bit more user-friendly; however, an example will be seen later (See: Figure 3-9).

Mini-Summary

- Each pitch is tested to see how loud it needs to be for you to just barely hear it. This is your threshold for each pitch.
- The hearing levels for the right ear are depicted with Os, and the left ear is depicted with Xs.

⊞Audiogram Alert!

On any given day, a person's hearing levels for pure tones can go up or down by about 5 dB. For example, on Monday a threshold at 1000 Hz could be 35; on Tuesday it could be 30, and on Wednesday it could be 40. This 5 dB-variability is normal, and can be explained by a variety of reasons. For example, if you are fatigued, your threshold could go down 5 dB because it takes a lot of concentration to keep listening to very soft tones. There's even evidence that diet plays a role in hearing. For example, the ear depends on a delicate balance of salt and potassium. If these levels are thrown off, hearing can be affected (see Chapter 8 Q&A #2).

While a 5 dB variability is not a concern, keep an eye on your first (baseline) hearing test. From one year to the next, a 5 dB shift might not seem unusual, but a 5 dB downward shift every year will have an impact on what hearing aids are selected for you.

"Give It To Me Straight, Doc—How Bad Is My Hearing?"

Figure 3-3 shows our three audiogram components with a complete pure tone hearing test. The Os and Xs are connected with lines to help the eye track the hearing levels across the pitches. But what does it all mean? This takes us to the next step in interpreting your audiogram.

Hearing levels can be described in a progression of loss: normal, mild, moderate, moderately severe, severe, or profound. These levels of loss are added to Figure 3-3. The hearing levels depicted here are typical for many patients. Both ears start off at normal levels in the low pitches, drop to a mild loss in the middle pitches, and then end with a moderate loss in the high pitches.

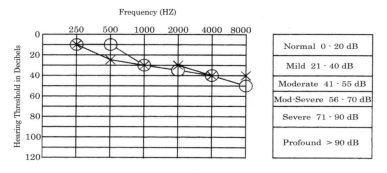

Figure 3-3: Mild to moderate hearing loss both ears.

Because there are different hearing levels (normal and also mild and moderate degrees of hearing loss) across the pitches, how would you describe this hearing loss?

Your hearing report would probably reveal close to what is written in the previous paragraph, but in conversation, you can accurately say this person has a mild to moderate hearing loss in the mid to high frequencies, both ears.

Figure 3-4 demonstrates how as the loudness increases, the hearing levels drop down the audiogram. In this example, the hearing loss we saw in Figure 3-3 has dropped about 10 to 45 dB, indicating moderate-to-severe hearing loss in both ears.

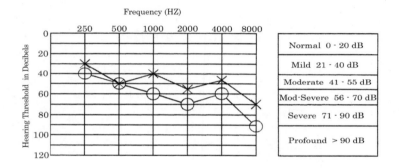

Figure 3-4: Moderate to severe hearing loss both ears.

By the way, in this chapter I am assuming that you are experiencing a hearing loss in both ears (called a bilateral loss). Occasionally, individuals have hearing loss only in one ear, with normal hearing in the other. This condition is called a unilateral (one-sided) hearing loss, and it presents unique challenges in localizing sound sources and listening in noise. Ask your hearing health professional for more information if you have a unilateral hearing loss.

Mini-Summary

- Hearing levels can be summarized with descriptors such as normal, mild, moderate, moderately severe, severe, and profound.
- These descriptors may need to be combined to describe all the pitches (from low, middle, and high) accurately.

- How you hear pure tones is directly related to how you hear speech—the ultimate question you want to answer. Your test may have included how soft you could hear speech (speech recognition threshold, reported in decibels). These results are often included on the same form as your audiogram.

⊞Audiogram Alert!

Occasionally, you will hear people use percentages to describe their hearing loss, as in "I was told I have a 50 percent loss in my right ear." There are two circumstances that could explain this kind of description. First, the American Medical Association developed a percentage system years ago to describe hearing loss, and occasionally physicians still use it. However, as you look at an audiogram, you can see that decibels do not translate into percentages, and the hearing levels for each pitch are not addressed at all. So the percentage system, while intending to be helpful, does not really tell you much, and could even be misleading.

The other explanation could be confusing with some audiological testing that *is* reported in percentages. After finding out how you heard pure tones, your hearing care professional may have also wanted to know how well you hear one-syllable words. This is necessary to understand your hearing difficulties, and was touched on in the previous chapter.

The Connection From Pure Tones to Speech Sounds

All along I have been saying that the pure tones by which you had been tested are related to how you hear and understand speech. Figure 3-5 is an audiogram with speech sounds superimposed over it. It shows how speech sounds are spread out in pitch. It has been noted that this shape vaguely resembles a banana, so it is often called the "speech banana."

Vowels are relatively low in pitch, while consonants that use voicing (for example, /l/, /m/, /n/) are in the middle range of pitches. "Voicing" means your voice helps produce the sound. To experience this, place your finger tips on your throat and hum a long "mmm." You will feel your throat vibrate. You are feeling your larynx or voice box move as air travels from your lungs to your mouth.

Many speech sounds are high in pitch (for example, /s / and /f/). These are produced without voicing, making them extremely soft as well as high-pitched. For example, put your upper teeth over your lower lip and gently blow through. This is the position for /f/. Without using your voice, try to blow harder, attempting to make the /f/ sound louder. You'll immediately notice that it cannot be done very well because the power for speech comes from your voice. The /f/ is voiceless. Now add your voice to it by humming through your lips in the same position. By doing this, you now no longer have an /f/ but a /v/ because you added vocalization, which will make this sound *much* easier to hear.

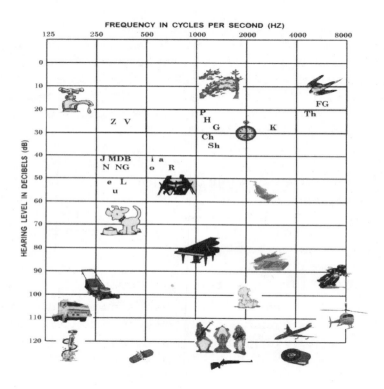

Figure 3-5: "Familiar Sounds" audiogram.

     All sounds for speech vibrate at different frequencies, which is how you differentiate speech sounds. Two of the highest consonant sounds in English are /f/ and /s/. Even a mild hearing loss in the high frequencies can make either sound inaudible. If you miss hearing so much as one sound in one word in a single thought, it can be enough to miss the entire message. This is why some sounds seem garbled or muffled. It may sound like someone is mumbling. This situation explains the observation made by many people with hearing loss: "I can hear you, I just can't understand you!" Not picking up some of the speech sounds will make speech hard to understand, although general speech activity can still be heard.

As hearing levels drop, more and more speech sounds become harder to hear. This is the information your hearing care professional is looking to assess in order to appropriately fit you with hearing aids—but it all starts with those pure tones.

⊞Audiogram Alert!

Your hearing care professional may have spent some time explaining your audiogram to you once the testing was completed. If you found it confusing, you may have felt too distracted or overwhelmed with the confirmation of having a hearing loss. Don't be discouraged! It's a lot of information to take in, and you should give yourself credit for getting this far in this chapter.

More Practice

The more audiograms you see, the more sense they make. Following are four additional audiograms to consider before we take a look at your own audiogram. Figure 3-6 shows normal hearing in both ears up to 2000 Hz. Hearing levels drop to a moderate loss at 4000 Hz, and then recover to a mild loss at 8000 Hz. This type of configuration usually suggests a history of excessive noise exposure. It is such a commonly observed configuration, it has its own name: "noise notch." A person with this kind of hearing loss is strongly advised to take every measure necessary to protect against further noise exposure. Without hearing protection, this hearing loss can drop more and more, and eventually affect the middle and high frequencies.

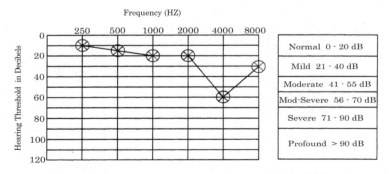

Figure 3-6: Hearing loss consistent with noise exposure.

Many hearing losses show gradual change from one frequency to the next, but some people have the kind of hearing loss shown in Figure 3-7. We see normal hearing in both ears through 1000 Hz, and then a dramatic, precipitous drop at 2000 Hz. Typically, 1500 Hz is not tested but because of the difference between 1000 and 2000, this information is important to collect. This audiogram represents a moderately severe to profound hearing loss in the mid to high frequencies, right ear worse than left.

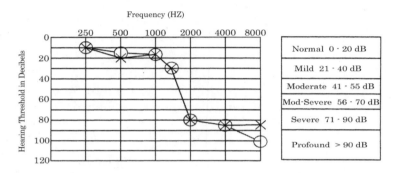

Figure 3-7: Normal hearing in low pitches with a severe precipitous drop.

In comparison, Figure 3-8 shows a severe-to-profound hearing loss in all the speech frequencies. No speech sounds produced at normal volume will be audible, although loud sounds in the environment might be barely heard.

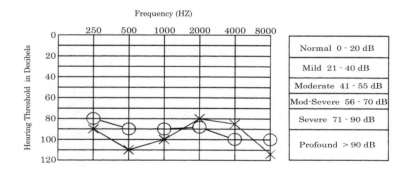

Figure 3-8: Severe to profound hearing loss both ears.

52

If you are a typical person with hearing loss, you have a sensorineural type of loss, meaning the sensory organ of hearing (the inner ear) is permanently losing its sensitivity. But hearing can also be temporarily affected by middle ear problems. These changes could be caused by severe head colds, allergies, damaged eardrums or other medical problems. This kind of hearing problem (called a conductive loss) will also be reflected in the audiogram, and we have one example here.

With its Os and Xs, Figure 3-9 indicates that a severe hearing loss exists in both ears in the low frequencies, recovering to a moderate hearing loss in the middle and high frequencies. However, when listening to pure tones with a bone oscillator (shown with bracket symbols), this person has better hearing levels in the low frequencies than indicated with headphones alone. Because of a middle ear problem, it is even harder than usual to hear low frequencies (note the poorer hearing levels). When a conductive loss is combined with a sensorineural loss, it is described as a *mixed loss*. Middle ear problems usually can be treated with medications or surgery. A person with an audiogram like one in Figure 3-9 will have better hearing if the conductive components are resolved (although a moderate sensorineural loss will remain in those lower frequencies).

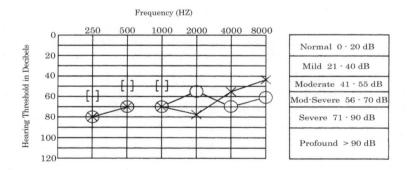

Figure 3-9: Moderate sensorineual hearing loss both ears, with additional middle ear (conductive) hearing loss in lower frequencies.

Now It's Your Turn!

To help translate this chapter into personally meaningful information, the following questions are presented. Please locate a copy of your audiogram and follow these easy steps:

1. Carefully transcribe your audiogram's Os and Xs onto the blank audiogram in Figure 3-1.
2. Connect all the Os with a straight line
3. Connect all the Xs with a straight line.
4. Now you want to find out how well you hear within the critical range of hearing for human speech. Find your hearing threshold at 500 Hz for the right ear by looking on the graph below 500 until you see the O.
5. What is the dB level? Write it in here: _____ dB.
6. Look at the notation to the right that reveals the range from *normal* to *profound*, and write what yours is: _____.
7. Do the same for 4000 Hz as you just did for 500 Hz.
8. What is the range from *normal* to *profound* for 4000 Hz? Write what yours is: _____.
9. What are the ranges where your hearing levels start and end (for example, "*moderate* to *severe*" or perhaps even "*mild*" across all frequencies)? _____.
10. For the right ear, you should now know the range of loss you have. You can now do the same for the left ear.
11. Left ear loss at 500 Hz is: _____.
12. Left ear loss at 4000 Hz is: _____.
13. Left ear range of loss at 500 Hz is: _____.
14. Left ear range of loss at 4000 Hz is: _____.
15. What is the final range of hearing for your left ear (for example, *mild* to *severe*)? _____.
16. Now locate one of the many audiograms among Figures 3-6 through 3-20 in this chapter that most resembles your own audiogram. An easy way to match this is by noting your hearing levels for one ear at a time. Observe your loss only at these four frequencies: 500, 1000, 2000 and 4000 Hz and determine the best match for one ear.
17. You can now read the interpretation for the audiogram you matched, as described in that Figure. Ask yourself, what speech sounds are you missing? (See: Figure 3-5 to find the answer to this question.) Are you a hearing aid candidate? What challenges lay ahead for you?
18. Repeat the match for the other ear if the hearing levels differ from the first ear's best match.

We've already briefly discussed Figures 3-6 through 3-9, so let's consider the remaining audiograms. If your audiogram closely resembles Figure 3-10, you have a hearing loss of some degree in the low and perhaps middle frequencies, and normal hearing in the higher ranges. This kind of hearing loss is often caused by health conditions such as diabetes, Meniere's Disease, or labyrinthitis (an inner ear infection described in Chapter 8 Q&A #6). You could be missing as much as 30 percent of speech information, and like all hearing loss configurations, you probably find it hard to understand people in noisy situations. Hearing aids (programmable or ideally digital) can help you hear better.

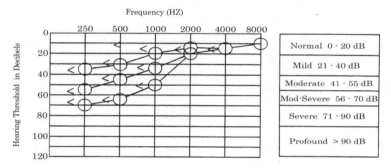

Figure 3-10: A variety of low frequency sensorineural hearing losses right ear only.

Keep in mind that the more normal your hearing across the frequency ranges, especially progressing into the higher ranges, the better you will function in your hearing world. If your audiogram closely resembles Figures 3-11, 3-12 or 3-13, you have a mild hearing loss at some of the tested frequencies. You could be missing up to 40% of speech, making it difficult to follow conversations, especially in noisy situations (restaurants, parties, etc.).

You will note that Figures 3-12 and 3-13 have hearing loss restricted to only the higher ranges. Figure 3-13 is limited to loss only in the uppermost range (furthest to the right on the audiogram). The latter indicates that someone with this loss may hear fairly well overall except when in the most challenging situations around noise or very soft female voices, and may not be the best candidate for hearing aids. Persons with audiograms similar to Figures 3-11 and 3-12 might well utilize hearing aids with only a minimum of power to pick up softer consonants that make speech clear.

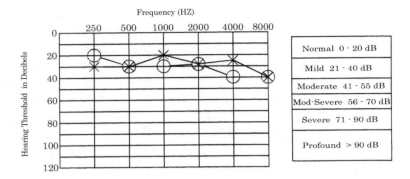

Figure 3-11: Mild hearing loss both ears all frequencies (flat mild loss).

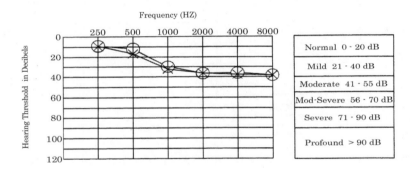

Figure 3-12: Mild mid-to-high frequency hearing loss both ears (with normal hearing in lows).

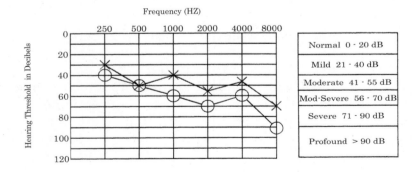

Figure 3-13: Normal hearing low and mid frequencies with a mild loss in the high frequencies.

If your audiogram closely resembles Figures 3-14, 3-15 or 3-16, you have a moderate hearing loss at some of the tested frequencies. However, depending on where your loss occurs in the frequency range, you will experience a different set of problems. Naturally, the further away you are from the conversation you are trying to hear, the more difficult it will be for anyone to understand.

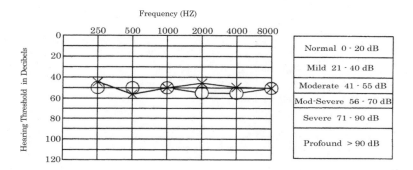

Figure 3-14: Moderate hearing loss in all frequencies (moderate flat loss) both ears.

Figure 3-14 indicates that with about equal loss across all tested frequencies, understanding almost all speech at five feet in a quiet room could prove challenging. For example, if your spouse was reading behind a newspaper, yet only five feet away, you will not have the advantage of speech cues and would likely miss most of what would be said.

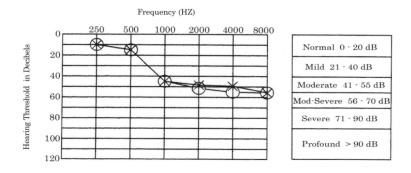

Figure 3-15: Moderate mid-to-high frequemcy hearing loss both ears with normal hearing in the lows.

On the other hand, if your loss is limited to only the high range (Figure 3-16), you are likely to do much better. As you have no doubt already noticed, noisy situations make hearing even more difficult. Many of these environmental intrusions you can control yourself, such as turning down the music or television. Hearing aids are especially helpful with these kinds of hearing losses since they greatly assist in bringing back the intelligibility of speech.

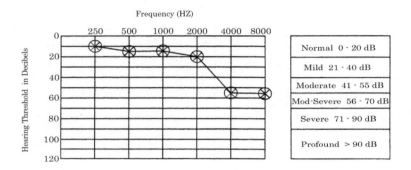

Figure 3-16: Normal hearing in low and mid frequencies, with a moderate loss in the high frequencies for both ears.

If your audiogram closely resembles Figure 3-17, you have a severe hearing loss across all frequencies. You already know that speech is not audible to you, and that hearing aids must be used in order to hear people and the sounds in your environment. The better your word discrimination ability under sound booth testing conditions *without hearing aids* the better your prognosis for benefit *with hearing aids.*

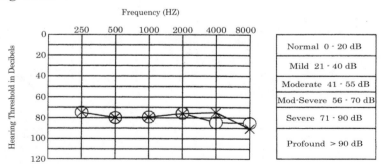

Figure 3-17: Severe hearing loss in all frequencies both ears.

If your audiogram resembles Figure 3-18, the configuration could reflect someone who spent a career around toxic levels of noise (compressors, hammers, drills, saws, etc.). You are hearing mostly vowels—lots of vocal energy with not much clarity. The intelligibility for speech (consonants) is at best very muffled. You are missing a considerable percentage of conversation and your use of hearing aids is both necessary and probably beneficial, especially if your word discrimination ability was tested and found to be good.

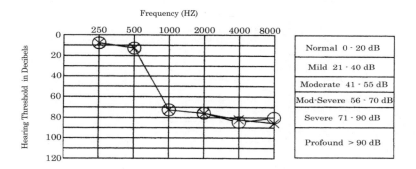

Figure 3-18: Severe mid-to-high frequency hearing loss both ears with normal low frequencies.

If your audiogram resembles Figure 3-19, your hearing levels are normal in the low and middle frequencies, but your high frequency hearing loss is severe. This audiogram includes threshold information at 3000 Hz, usually tested when the shift between 2000 and 4000 is so significant. This allows for a more accurate picture of the audiogram, and your potential hearing challenges. In this case, higher frequency consonants will be very difficult to hear (such as /f/, /k/, /s/ or /th/) and in the presence of some background noise, may even be wiped out. This type of audiogram has been seen in people who have done extensive firearms training without hearing protection for years, usually with the same or similar caliber weapon. Hearing aids can provide emphasis to the high frequencies and fill in much of what you are missing.

If your audiogram resembles Figure 3-20, you are already aware that you experience a profound loss in all frequencies. Powerful hearing aids are probably something you've been wearing for some time in order to receive as much auditory information as possible from speech and environmental sounds. If you are new to hearing aids with this kind of loss, you might consider exploring other options, such as a cochlear implant or an expanded system of assistive devices. Implants are increasingly viable options for many patients, but candidacy criteria must be discussed with your physician and hearing care professional. Assistive devices are helpful to all persons with hearing loss, and the more severe the loss, the more helpful the devices.

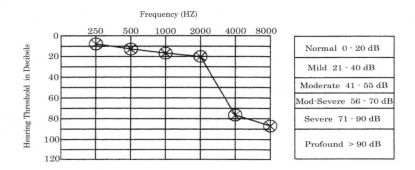

Figure 3-19: Normal hearing in mid and low frequencies with a severe hearing loss in the high frequencies both ears.

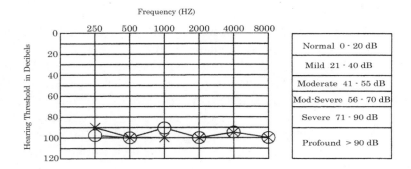

Figure 3-20: Profound hearing loss in all frequencies both ears.

Audiograms May Not Be The Whole Story

We have spent considerable time reviewing how hearing levels are objectively measured and recorded. One final point must be mentioned: an audiogram does not always predict how you experience life. Two people can have identical audiograms but have very different reactions to the stresses and problems hearing loss causes. One person with mild to moderate hearing loss may experience a great deal of difficulty, while another person with the same hearing loss (or worse) may have fewer challenges.

Why would this be?

It seems to boil down to our individuality—the uniqueness that identifies each of us for who we are: our personality type, our perception of ourselves, our view of the world, and even our desire or motivation to communicate. A housebound reclusive person may be less likely to pursue hearing aids than an extroverted individual who continually engages with people to experience the joys of life. The truth is that some of us do not care to hear. Others are driven to solve their hearing problem.

Your hearing care professional would not assume that by knowing your audiogram, he or she also knows your listening challenges. Let your practitioner know your hearing needs and expectations so you can receive the maximum benefit with the technology now available to you. Help fill in the information that the audiogram cannot.

CHAPTER FOUR
Hearing Aids Positively Improve Your Quality of Life

Sergei Kochkin, Ph.D.

Dr. Kochkin is a Director of Market Development & Market Research at Knowles Electronics and past member of the Board of Directors of the Better Hearing Institute in Washington, D.C. He has published more than 50 papers on the hearing aid market and conducted customer satisfaction research on more than 25,000 hearing aid owners. He holds a Doctorate in psychology, an MBA in marketing, a Masters of Science in counseling and guidance and a BA in physical anthropology and archeology. Dr. Kochkin also maintains an interest in ancient cultures, comparative religion and meditation.

The number one reason why people purchase their first hearing aids is they recognize their hearing has worsened. The second reason is pressure from family members who are negatively impacted by the individual's hearing loss. As you know by now, hearing loss occurs gradually. By the time you recognize a need for hearing aids, your quality of life may have deteriorated unnecessarily. The average first-time hearing aid wearer is close to 70 years of age, despite the fact that the majority (65 percent) of people with hearing loss are below the age of 65; and nearly half of all people with hearing loss are below the age of 55.

For the vast majority of individuals who have decided to wait to purchase hearing aids *(78 percent of all people who admit to hearing loss),* I suspect that while they may be aware their hearing loss has deteriorated, they delay hearing aid purchases under the excuses: *"my hearing loss is not bad enough yet; I can get by without them; my hearing loss is mild."* A large number of people wait 15 years or more from the point when they first recognize they have a hearing loss to when they purchase their first hearing aids. This is a tragedy since they might not be aware of the impact this delayed decision has had on their life and the lives of their family, friends and associates.

The literature presents a compelling story for the social, psychological, cognitive and health effects of hearing loss. Impaired hearing results in distorted or incomplete communication leading to greater isolation and withdrawal and therefore lower sensory input.

In turn, the individuals life space and social life becomes restricted. One would logically think that a constricted life would negatively impact the psychosocial well-being of people with hearing loss.

Dr. Carmen presented a number of emotional issues in Chapter One surrounding hearing loss. Here's a quick review, with some additional ones. The literature indicates that hearing loss is associated with: embarrassment, fatigue, irritability, tension and stress, anger, avoidance of social activities, withdrawal from social situations, depression, negativism, danger to personal safety, rejection by others, reduced general health, loneliness, social isolation, less alertness to the environment, impaired memory, less adaptability to learning new tasks, paranoia, reduced coping skills, and reduced overall psychological health. For those who are still in the work force, uncorrected hearing loss must have a negative impact on overall job effectiveness, promotion and perhaps lifelong earning power. We think few would disagree that uncorrected hearing loss per se is a serious issue.

Prior Experimental Evidence that Hearing Aids Improve Quality of Life

An effective human being is an effective communicator; optimized hearing is critical to effective communication. Modern hearing aids improve speech intelligibility and therefore communication. The benefits of hearing aids *(audiologically defined as improved speech intelligibility)* have been demonstrated in rigorous scientific research.[1] It would seem that if one could improve speech intelligibility by correcting for impaired hearing, that one should observe improvements in the social, emotional, psychological and physical functioning of the person with the hearing loss. To my knowledge there have only been a few studies to date comparing hearing aid owners and non-owners with known hearing loss. The majority of studies had small sample sizes and in general tended to confine themselves to U.S. male veterans. Let me first share these results with you before describing the exciting findings of a very large U.S. study I conducted in collaboration with the National Council on Aging in 1999 (with publication in January 2000).[2]

Harless and McConnell[3] demonstrated that 68 hearing aid wearers had significantly higher self-concepts compared to a matched group of individuals who did not wear hearing aids. Dye and Peak[4] studied 58 male veterans pre and post hearing aid fitting and found significant improvement on memory tests. In the most rigorous controlled study to date, Mulrow, Aguilar and Endicott[5] studied 122 male veterans and 72 patients from primary care clinics. Half were randomly chosen and fit with hearing aids while the other half were not. After four months compared to the control group, the researchers found significant improvements in the hearing aid wearers on emotional and social effects of hearing handicap, perceived communication difficulties, cognitive functioning, and depression.

In addition, the same researchers in a follow-up study[6] published in 1992 demonstrated that the quality of life changes were sustainable over at least a year. Bridges and Bentler[7] determined in a study of 251 subjects comprised of normal hearing elderly individuals with hearing aids, and individuals with unaided hearing loss, that hearing aid wearers had less depression and higher quality of life scores compared to their unaided counterparts.

Finally, in a pre-post study *(that is the person was studied before and after a hearing aid fitting)* with 20 subjects, Crandall[8] demonstrated after three months of hearing aid use that functional health status improved significantly for hearing aid wearers.

Research on the Positive Impact of Hearing Aids on Quality of Life

I would now like to share with you the results of the largest study in the world conducted on the impact of hearing aids on quality of life. After reading this, I hope you agree that hearing aids when successfully fit to your unique audiological needs, have the potential to literally transform your life.

Utilizing the famous National Family Opinion Panel (NFO) in 1997, I mailed a short screening survey to 80,000 panel members to find a representative sample of people with hearing loss in the United States. This short survey helped identify nearly 15,000 people with self-admitted hearing loss. The response rate to the screening survey was 65 percent. Since 1989, I have conducted research in this manner on more than 25,000 people with hearing loss and published these findings under the generic name "MarkeTrak." Working with the National Council on Aging, a sample of 3,000 individuals with hearing loss ages 50 and over were randomly drawn from the MarkeTrak hearing loss panel. Equal samples of 1,500 hearing aid owners and non-owners were drawn from the panel. What is unique about this study is that people with hearing loss as well as their significant other (usually the spouse) were studied.

Extensive questionnaires were sent to both the person with the hearing loss and the spouse or family member. The number of questions was 300 and 150 respectively. The comprehensive survey covered a myriad of topics including: self and family assessment of hearing loss, psychological well-being, social impact of hearing loss, quality of relationships, life satisfaction, general health, self and family perceptions of benefit of hearing aids *(wearers only)*, reasons for purchasing hearing aids *(wearers only)*, reasons for not purchasing hearing aids *(non-wearers only)*, and attitudes toward hearing health and hearing aids. In addition, a number of personality scales, which were deemed relevant to this study, were included in the survey.

After analyzing the returned surveys for usability (e.g. minimal missing information, hearing aid owners who wear their hearing instruments) the final sample sizes for respondents with hearing loss and family members were reduced to 2,069 and 1,710 respectively. Thus, this study involved nearly 4,000 people.

It was my goal to determine if hearing aids had an impact on hearing loss independent of the degree of hearing loss. In other words, do people with mild hearing loss derive as much benefit as individuals with more serious hearing losses? As part of the research design, in addition to quality of life items, a paper and pencil assessment of hearing loss was administered with the anticipation that the results of this assessment would be used to control for hearing loss when comparing the quality of life of hearing aid wearers and non-wearers.

The key hearing assessment tool used was the *Five Minute Hearing Test* (FMHT) by the American Academy of Otolaryngology-Head and Neck Surgery. The FMHT is a fifteen-question test measuring self-perceived hearing difficulty in a number of listening situations (e.g. telephone, multiple speakers, television, noisy situations, reverberant rooms) as well as self-assessments of some signs of hearing loss (e.g. people mumble, inappropriate responses, strain to hear, avoid social situations). Previous research has determined that the FMHT is significantly correlated with objective audiological hearing loss measures.

Based on hearing difficulty scores, all subjects in this study were grouped into five equal size groups (20 percent each—called quintiles). These ranged from quintile 1 (the 20 percent of respondents with the mildest hearing loss as measured by the FMHT) to quintile 5 (the 20 percent with the greatest hearing loss). The quintile system was utilized for all analysis as a means of controlling for differences in hearing loss between the hearing aid wearer and non-wearer samples. The use of these quintiles allowed us to achieve more valid comparisons between samples of hearing aid wearers and non-wearers.

If we were to simply compare responses of all hearing aid wearers with those of all non-wearers, without regard to degree of hearing loss, the findings would have been misleading, and even erroneous. For example, it is widely known that incidence and degree of depression have been found to increase with severity of hearing loss. Thus, even if people with severe hearing loss experience reduced depression after getting hearing aids, they might still report more depression than non-wearers overall, since hearing aid wearers tend to have more severe hearing loss. However, when hearing aid wearers are matched with non-wearers in the same quintile (non-wearers having a fairly similar degree of hearing loss), the differences between them better reflect the potential impact of the hearing aids rather than the effect of their degree of hearing loss.

While we have no audiological basis for labeling hearing loss associated with each quintile group, we did find an excellent correlation between self-perceived loss (e.g. mild to profound hearing loss) and the FMHT test. As we discuss the findings of this study with respect to the five hearing loss groups, it's appropriate to consider people in quintile hearing loss groups 1, 3 and 5 as having respectively a "mild," "moderate," and "severe /profound" hearing loss; group 2 is between mild and moderate hearing loss while group 4 should be viewed as between moderate and severe hearing loss.

Research Findings

We will now systematically evaluate the impact that hearing aids have on quality of life. This will be done by comparing the responses of hearing aid wearers and non-wearers while controlling for hearing loss. As you evaluate the impressive findings below keep in mind the following:

- the devastating impact of hearing loss on quality of life is well-documented;
- quality of life is primarily impacted by the fact that uncorrected hearing loss results in reduced speech intelligibility;
- hearing aids when fitted correctly improve speech intelligibility and therefore can restore your ability to function more effectively in life.

Demographics and Household Income

It should be recognized that in most respects the five hearing loss groups were well matched on key demographics: gender, marital status, employment status, and age. A striking trend was discovered when evaluating household income by level of hearing loss. Income is significantly related to both hearing loss and hearing aid usage. Figure 4-1 shows there was close to an $8,000 difference between those with mild hearing loss (quintile 1) and those with profound hearing loss (quintile 5). Note that income drops significantly only for severe to profound hearing loss groups (4 and 5—the top 40 percent of individuals with hearing loss).

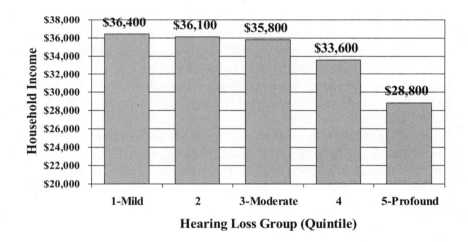

Figure 4-1: Household income is related to severity of hearing loss.

Compared to non-wearers, there was a $13,000 a year difference between the mild and profound hearing loss groups. The differential for hearing aid wearers was much less severe ($7,000). Hearing aids appeared to have a positive impact on household income, but only for individuals whose hearing loss was in the higher 60 percent (moderate-profound). People with a moderate to profound hearing loss, who did not use hearing aids, on average, experienced household incomes $5000-$6000 less than their counterparts who did use hearing aids. This is despite the fact that the higher hearing loss non-wearer groups tended to be employed slightly more often.

Hearing aid wearers also reported that they have plenty of discretionary income more often than non-wearers. For example, 22 percent of group 5 (profound hearing loss) hearing aid wearers reported they had plenty of discretionary income compared to only 8 percent of non-wearers. The discretionary income differential for samples with more severe hearing loss was a likely cause of the lower earning power. Because of higher hearing disability levels, communication is probably impacted, resulting in lower income and therefore less earning power. Finding a solution to their hearing loss is exacerbated for these groups, in that lower earning power means that the respondent was less likely to be able to afford a hearing aid to correct the hearing loss.

Activity Level

We asked respondents to indicate the extent (times per month) to which they engaged in thirteen activities in a typical month. Six of the activities were solitary in nature while seven involved other people. Total solitary and social activity scores were calculated. Hearing aid wearers were shown to have the same level of solitary activity as non-wearers. However, hearing aid wearers were more likely to engage in activities involving other people. They were shown to have significantly higher participation in three to four of the seven activities measured. Four out of five quintile hearing aid wearer groups indicated they participated more in organized social activities while three out of five of the hearing loss groups reported they were more likely to attend senior centers if they were hearing aid wearers. The most serious hearing loss group (quintile 5) reported greater participation in four out of the seven activities if they were hearing aid wearers.

Interpersonal relations

The survey asked 12 questions concerning the respondents' quality of interpersonal relationships with their family using a four-point scale. Twelve questions concerned negativity (e.g. arguments, tenseness, criticism) in the relationship. We found that interpersonal warmth in relationships significantly declined as hearing loss worsened. Hearing aid wearers in quintiles 1-3 (mild to moderate) were shown to have significantly greater interpersonal warmth in their relationships than their non-wearer counterparts. Also, significant reductions in negativity in family relationships appeared to be associated with hearing aid usage in quintiles 1 and 2—the hearing loss groups with the mildest hearing disability.

Social Effects

Forty-seven items in the survey assessed the social impact of hearing loss and hearing aid usage. The majority of the items were scored on a five-point scale taking the values "strongly agree" to "strongly disagree." We also assessed average monthly contact with family and friends by phone and in person.

The stigma of hearing loss was shown to increase as hearing loss increased. All five non-wearer groups reported they would be embarrassed or self-conscious if they wore hearing aids, while all five wearer groups reported lower stigmatization with hearing aids. We are not concluding, of course, that usage of hearing aids would lead to reduced stigma; most likely hearing aid wearers have resolved their concerns about the stigma associated with hearing aid usage more so than their non-wearer counterparts.

As hearing loss increased, respondents were more likely to overcompensate for hearing loss by pretending that they heard what people said, by avoiding telling people to repeat themselves, by avoiding asking other people to help them with their hearing problem, by engaging in compensatory activities such as speechreading, or by defensively talking too much to cover up the fact that they could not hear well.

All five hearing aid wearer groups reported significantly lower overcompensation scores. The greater the hearing loss, the greater was the likelihood that respondents reported they were the target of discrimination. The greater the hearing loss, the greater the likelihood that respondents with more serious hearing losses were accused of hearing only what they wanted to hear, found themselves the subject of conversation behind their backs, were told to "forget it" when frustrated family members were not heard the first time, and so on. All hearing loss groups except quintile 1 (the mildest hearing loss) reported significant reductions in discriminatory behaviors, if they were hearing aid wearers.

We found a strong relationship between hearing loss and family member concerns of safety (e.g. cannot hear warning signs, instructions from doctor, made a serious mistake, not safe to be alone) as well as significant differences between hearing aid wearers and non-wearers. Respondents also agreed that safety concerns increased as hearing loss increased.

The data however, indicated that safety concerns were significantly higher among hearing aid wearers than non-wearers in quintiles 1-3. Perhaps the realization that mistakes were being made or that unaided hearing loss could result in possible injury, motivated the current hearing aid owner to purchase hearing aids. This explanation is consistent with the findings from previous MarkeTrak research, which indicated that the number one motivation to purchase hearing aids was "the realization that their hearing loss was getting worse."

There were a number of social effects that were correlated with hearing loss but were not impacted by hearing aid usage. These were negative effects on the family (e.g., "I find it exhausting to cope with their needs"), family accommodations to the individual with hearing loss (e.g., "I have to use signs and gestures a lot of the time"), rejection of the person with hearing loss (e.g., "They tend to get left out of social activities because of their hearing loss"), and withdrawal (e.g., "They tend to withdraw from social activities where communication is difficult"). In addition, hearing aid usage was not associated with increased phone or in-person contact with family or friends.

The Emotional Effects

Eighty items in the survey dealt with the emotional aspects of hearing loss. All five hearing aid wearer groups scored significantly lower in their self-ratings of emotional instability. In agreement with their family members, they were less likely to be tense, insecure, unstable, nervous, discontent, temperamental, and less likely to display negative emotions or traits. Four of the five hearing aid wearer groups reported significantly reduced tendencies to exhibit anger (e.g., "I sometimes get angry when I think about my hearing") and frustration (e.g., "I get discouraged because of my hearing loss"). In agreement, family members observed significantly less anger and frustration in all five hearing aid wearer groups.

The average reduction in depression associated with hearing aid usage across all five groups was 36 percent. All five hearing aid wearer groups reported significantly *lower* depressive symptoms (e.g., tired, insomniac, thinking of death) while four of the five hearing aid wearer groups (quintiles 1-4) reported a significantly lower incidence of depression within the last 12 months compared to their non-wearer counterparts.

Hearing aid wearers in quintiles 2-4 reported significantly

lower paranoid feelings (e.g., "I am often blamed for things that are just not my fault"). Not surprisingly, in agreement with family members, all five non-wearer groups scored higher on denial when compared to hearing aid wearers (e.g., "I don't think my hearing loss is as bad as people have told me").

Family members and respondents were asked to indicate if the person with the hearing loss exhibited anxiety, tenseness or if they worried for a continuous period of four weeks in the previous year. In addition, they were asked to indicate if they experienced anxiety symptoms (e.g., keyed up or on edge, heart pounding or racing, easily tired, trouble falling asleep). Three of the five non-wearer groups (1, 3, 5) exhibited higher anxiety symptoms. In addition, three of the five non-wearer groups (1, 2, 5) exhibited more social phobias than non-wearers of hearing aids. Clearly, the reduction in phobia and anxiety associated with hearing aid usage is more pronounced in individuals with serious to profound hearing losses (Quintile 5).

Factors *not* appreciably impacted by hearing aid usage in this study were: sense of independence (e.g., burden on family, answering for the person with hearing loss) and overall satisfaction with life. Although not as conclusive as some of the previous factors, non-wearers reported that they were more self-critical (e.g., "I dwell on my mistakes more than I should") and had lower self-esteem (e.g., "All in all, I'm inclined to feel that I am a failure"). Hearing loss was found to be highly correlated with self-criticism. There is also some evidence, though not as strong as other correlates of hearing aid use, that non-wearers were more critical of themselves (Quintiles 1, 3, 5).

Personality Assessment

Seventy-nine items were devoted to miscellaneous personality scales in addition to the personality measures under emotional and social effects. All of the personality scales used in this study are published scales. Family members indicated that the respondents' cognitive/mental state (e.g., they appear confused, disoriented or unable to concentrate) was affected by their hearing loss, primarily if the hearing loss was "severe" to "profound" (groups 4 and 5). In this study, impressive improvements in family perceptions of the persons' mental and intellectual state were observed if the individual had a severe to profound hearing loss (groups 4 and 5 only). Non-wearers were more likely to be viewed as being confused, disoriented, non-caring, arrogant, inattentive, and virtually "living in a world of their own."

Previously we indicated that there were no significant differences in measures of "withdrawal" between aided and unaided subjects. This finding is contrary to the literature. However, family members did report that non-wearers in three of five groups (1,4, 5) were more introverted as evidenced by greater likelihood of being private, passive, shy, quiet, easily embarrassed, etc. Moderate to severe hearing loss non-wearers (quintiles 3-5) were shown to score higher on a personality variable called "external locus of control." This means they were more likely to believe that events external to them control their lives. In other words, they felt less in control of their own lives. On the other hand, hearing aid wearers felt they were more in control of their lives and less a victim of fate.

Health Impact

The survey asked six generic questions on self-perceptions of health, prevalence of pain and the extent to which the respondent believed that hearing loss impacted their general health. In addition, from a list of 28 health problems, respondents indicated whether they experienced that health problem and the extent to which the problem interfered with their activities.

Overall assessment of health (including absence of pain) appeared to decline as a function of hearing loss with further deterioration of health associated with non-usage of hearing aids for the three most serious hearing loss groups (quintiles 3-5). Three of the five hearing aid wearer groups (quintiles 1, 3, 5) reported significantly better health compared to their non-wearer counterparts. The lowest self-rating of overall health was the non-wearer group in quintile 5 (profound hearing loss). Nonetheless, our research determined there was no consistent evidence that hearing aid usage is associated with reductions in arthritis, high blood pressure, heart problems or other serious disease states.

Perceived Benefit of Hearing Aids

As a validation check on our comparisons of hearing aid wearers and non-wearers, both respondents and their family members were asked to rate changes they observed in 16 areas of their life that they believed were due to the respondent using hearing aids. Total findings are shown in Figure 4-2. In general, for nearly all quality of life areas assessed, the observed improvements were positively related to degree of hearing loss. Family members in nearly every comparison observed greater improvements in the respondent.

The top three areas of observed improvement for both respondents and family members were *relationships at home, feelings about self* and *life overall*. The most impressive improvements were observed in quintile 5 (profound hearing loss) in that 11 of 16 lifestyle areas were rated as improved by at least 50 percent of the respondents or family members.

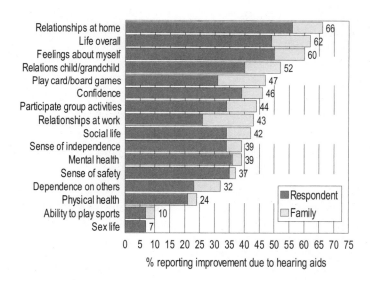

Figure 4-2: Percent of hearing aid owners and their family members reporting improvement in their quality of life in 16 areas due to hearing aids. In nearly all cases, family members report improvements due to hearing aids than hearing instrument wearers.

Conclusions and Discussion

The results for this study are impressive. Hearing aids clearly are associated with impressive improvements in the social, emotional, psychological, and physical well-being of people with hearing loss in all hearing loss categories from mild to severe. As such, these findings clearly provide strong evidence for the *value of hearing aids* in improving the quality of life in people with hearing loss. Specifically, hearing aid usage is positively related to the following quality of life issues:

- greater earning power (especially the more severe hearing losses)
- improved interpersonal relationships (especially for mild-moderate losses) including greater intimacy and lessening of negative dysfunctional communication
- reduction in discrimination toward the person with the hearing loss
- reduction in difficulty associated with communication (primarily severe to profound hearing losses)
- reduction in hearing loss compensation behaviors
- reduction in anger and frustration
- reduction in the incidence of depression and depressive symptoms
- enhanced emotional stability
- reduction in paranoid feelings
- reduced anxiety symptoms
- reduced social phobias (primarily severely impaired subjects)
- improved sense of control in your life
- reduced self-criticism
- improved cognitive functioning (primarily severe to profound hearing loss)
- improved health status and less incidence of pain
- enhanced group social activity

In this study, both respondents and their family members were asked to independently rate the extent to which they believed their life was specifically improved due to hearing aids. All hearing loss groups from mild to profound reported significant improvements in nearly every area measured:

- relationships at home and with family
- feelings about self
- life overall
- mental health
- social life
- emotional health
- physical health

Short of stating definite causality, the evidence is quite compelling and perhaps suggestive of causality for the following reasons:

74

1. The sample, the largest of its kind, is nationally representative of hearing loss subjects ages 50 and over. Thus, we need not be concerned with spurious findings due to sampling methodology.
2. Many of the findings held up across all hearing loss quintiles from mild to profound.
3. The specific findings were corroborated within the study. That is, we noted significant differences between wearers and non-wearers. Also, at the end of the survey we asked respondents and their family members to specifically indicate if their life was improved as a result of wearing hearing aids in 16 quality of life areas. Both respondents and their family members indicated significant benefit due to hearing aids in most areas measured.
4. The differential efficacy between the 16 quality of life parameters noted by respondents and their family members (from a low of 4 percent to high of 74 percent improvements) indicates that a positive halo or acquiescence did not exist in this sample of respondents.
5. The survey findings are correlated well with other studies, especially the randomized control studies and pre-post hearing aid fitting studies among smaller, more narrowly defined samples.
6. The findings are consistent with the literature on factors impacting hearing loss; that is, the theoretical improvements that should occur if hearing loss is alleviated.
7. The findings are consistent with the observations of clinicians and dispensers of hearing aids.

A Call to Action

Dr. Firman of the National Council On Aging stated in his speech to the media in the summer of 1999, "This study debunks the myth that untreated hearing loss...is a harmless condition."[9]

In focus groups conducted with physicians, the prevalent view is that hearing loss is "only" a quality of life issue. I would agree if one defined quality of life as "greater enjoyment of music." But the literature and this study clearly demonstrate that hearing loss is associated with physical, emotional, mental, and social well-being. Depression, anxiety, emotional instability, phobias, withdrawal, isolation, lessened health status, lower self-esteem, and so forth, are not "just quality of life issues." For some people, uncorrected hearing loss is a "life and death issue."

I believe that this study challenges every segment of society to comprehend the devastating impact of hearing loss on individuals and their families as well as the positive possibilities associated with hearing aid usage. We need to help physicians recognize hearing loss for the important health issue that it is. We need to help those with hearing loss who are currently in denial about their impairment, to understand the impact their hearing has on their life as well as that of their loved ones. We need to assure that hearing aids are recognized in society not just for their treatment of hearing loss, but also as a potential contributing factor to the successful resolution of other medical, emotional, social and psychological conditions.

I believe this study also demonstrates for the first time that individuals with even a mild hearing loss can experience dramatic improvements in their quality of life. This finding is significant because I believe the challenge is to demonstrate to "baby-boomers" (ages 45-59) with emerging hearing losses that hearing aids offer something to them of value early on in their lives, and that they do not need to wait until retirement to receive the benefits of enhanced hearing.

So if you are one of those people with a mild, moderate or severe hearing loss, who is sitting on the fence, consider all the benefits of hearing aids described above. I challenge you to name another product, which holds such great potential to positively change so many lives.

Editor's Note: The full research project this chapter is based on including detailed references, charts and figures are available at www.hearingreview.com.

References

1. Larson V.D., et. al. (17 other authors). Efficacy of Three Commonly Used Hearing Aid Circuits, JAMA 284(14):1806-1813, 2000.
2. Kochkin S and Rogin C. Quantifying the obvious: the impact of hearing aids on quality of life. The Hearing Review 7(1): 8-34, 2000.
3. Harless E and McConnell F. Effects of hearing aid use on self-concept in older persons. Journal of Speech and Hearing Disorders 47:305-309, 1982.

4. Dye C and Peak M. Influence on amplification on the psychological functioning of older adults with neurosensory hearing loss. Journal of the Academy of Rehabilitation Audiology 16:210-220,1983.

5. Mulrow C, Aguilar C, Endicott J, et al. Quality of life changes and hearing impairment. Annals of Internal Medicine 113(3):188-194, 1990.

6. Mulrow C, Tuley M and Aguilar C. Sustained benefits of hearing aids. Journal of Speech and Hearing Research 35:1402-1405,1992.

7. Bridges J and Bentler R. Relating hearing aid use to well-being among older adults. The Hearing Journal 51(7):39-44,1998.

8. Crandell C. Hearing aids: their effects on functional health status. The Hearing Journal 51(2):2-6,1998.

9. Firman J. Speech to the media on May 26, 1999 based on NCOA study National Council on the Aging (NCOA). The Impact of Untreated Hearing Loss in Older Americans. Conducted by the Seniors Research Group. Supported through a grant from the Hearing Industries Association. Preliminary report, December 28, 1998. Actual press release can be seen at www.ncoa.org.

CHAPTER FIVE
The Leap
From Hearing Loss to Hearing Aids
Barbara E. Weinstein, Ph.D.

Dr. Weinstein is a Professor of Audiology at Lehman College, City University of New York (CUNY), and is a member of the doctoral faculty at the Graduate School and University Center, CUNY. She is a Fellow of the American Speech-Language-Hearing Association, and is the recipient of the 1996 Distinguished Clinical Achievement Award from the New York State Speech-Language-Hearing Association. Dr. Weinstein is the author of a text titled: *Geriatric Audiology* and has edited several books on hearing loss in the elderly. She is the co-author of the Hearing Handicap Inventory for Adults and the Elderly and has authored over 50 manuscripts on hearing loss and hearing aids in adults.

Responses to questionnaires that assess activity limitations and participation levels are quite important as they assist the hearing care professional in understanding the functional effects of a chronic condition such as hearing impairment. Answers to items comprising the Hearing Handicap Inventory (HHI) can help you and your hearing care provider better understand how hearing impairment interferes with a range of activities considered integral in your daily life.

As is apparent from the items shown in Tables 5-I and 5-II, responses to the questionnaires reveal perceptions of auditory and non-auditory difficulties (e.g. such as embarrassment, frustration) resulting from diminished auditory capacity. To reiterate, these self-report questionnaires provide information from your perspective about problems associated with hearing impairment. Once your hearing professional has a feel for the social and emotional consequences of your hearing loss and the impact of these changes on your independence and quality of life, it can be determined if you are a candidate for hearing aids or if you are obtaining adequate benefit from hearing aids.

Hearing Handicap Inventories

The 10-item screening (symbolized by "-S") versions of the Hearing Handicap Inventory for Adults (HHIA-S) or for the Elderly

(HHIE-S) have gained widespread acceptance among physicians, nurses, nurse practitioners, and audiologists. The HHIE-S (Table 5-I) was standardized on adults over 65 years of age and is hence more appropriate for them. The HHIA-S, shown in Table 5-III is primarily for individuals under 65 years of age. With the exception of three items, the emotions and situations sampled are identical. The HHIE-SP/HHIA-SP (Table 5-II), where SP is short for spouse, is a companion version that enables the hearing care practitioner to elicit responses from a spouse regarding the effects of hearing loss. Evident from the items comprising the questionnaires, responses can pinpoint the social and emotional consequences of your hearing impairment as perceived by you and a significant other.

Each of the questionnaires can be completed at home using paper and pencil, by computer-assisted presentation with links to audiologists in all 50 states (www.phd.msu.edu/hearing), or by face-to-face administration with a professional asking the questions. Each form of administration has its advantages and disadvantages, but the bottom line is what is most convenient for the person with hearing impairment. Each of the scales consists of two types of questions, namely social (S) and emotional (E). The five social questions attempt to isolate the self-perceived difficulties in a given situation whereas the five emotional questions assess anxiety, frustration, and overall sense of handicap that is attributed to hearing loss.

You merely check or answer "Yes" if you experience difficulty in the situation described; "Sometimes" if you experience occasional difficulty in the given situation; or "No" if you rarely or never experience the problem. A score of "4" is awarded each Yes response, a score of "2" each Sometimes response, and a score of "0" for each No response. Points for each of the 10 items are added up and total scores can range from 0 to 40. The higher the number, the greater is the problem of hearing loss. A score of 0-10 indicates that the hearing impairment is not interfering with your daily life. The average score for new hearing aid wearers on the screening versions of the HHIE is about 18.

A score of 10 or greater signifies the necessity for referral to a hearing healthcare professional. More specifically, scores of 0-8 signify *no handicap;* scores of 10-22 signify *a mild to moderate handicap;* and scores of 24-40 suggest significant *self-perceived handicap.*

Table 5-I: Hearing Handicap Inventory for the Elderly —Screening [HHIE-S]

INSTRUCTIONS: The purpose of this questionnaire is to identify the problems your hearing loss may be causing you. Answer YES, SOMETIMES, or NO for each question. To obtain a total score, add up the "yes" (4 points each), "sometimes" (2 points each), and "no" (0 points) responses. If your score is greater than 10, a hearing test is recommended.

Yes	Sometimes	No
4	2	0

E1 Does a hearing problem cause you to feel embarrassed when you meet new people?

E2 Does a hearing problem cause you to feel frustrated when talking to members of your family?

S1 Do you have difficulty hearing when someone speaks in a whisper?

E3 Do you feel handicapped by a hearing problem?

S2 Does a hearing problem cause you difficulty when visiting friends, relatives or neighbors?

S3 Does a hearing problem cause you to attend religious services less often than you would like?

E4 Does a hearing problem cause you to have arguments with family members?

S4 Does a hearing problem cause you difficulty when listening to TV or radio?

E5 Do you feel that any difficulty with your hearing limits or hampers your personal or social life?

S5 Does a hearing problem cause you difficulty when in a restaurant with relatives or friends?

Table 5-II: Hearing Handicap Inventory for the Elderly
—Screening [HHIE-SP]

INSTRUCTIONS: The purpose of this questionnaire is to identify the problems the hearing loss may be causing your spouse. Answer YES, SOMETIMES, or NO for each question. To obtain a total score, add up the "yes" (4 points each), "sometimes" (2 points each), and "no" (0 points) responses. If your score is greater than 10, a hearing test is recommended. SP=spouse.

Yes	Sometimes	No
4	2	0

E1 Does a hearing problem cause your SP to feel embarrassed when meeting new people?

E2 Does a hearing problem cause your SP to feel frustrated when talking to members of your family?

S1 Does your SP have difficulty hearing when someone speaks in a whisper?

E3 Does your SP feel handicapped by a hearing problem?

S2 Does a hearing problem cause your SP difficulty when visiting friends, relatives or neighbors?

S3 Does a hearing problem cause your SP to attend religious services less often than you would like?

E4 Does a hearing problem cause your SP to have arguments with family members?

S4 Does a hearing problem cause your SP difficulty when listening to TV or radio?

E5 Do you feel that any difficulty with hearing limits or hampers your SP's personal or social life?

S5 Does a hearing problem cause your SP difficulty when in a restaurant with relatives or friends?

Table 5-III: Hearing Handicap Inventory for Adult —Screening [HHIA-S]

INSTRUCTIONS: The purpose of this questionnaire is to identify the problems your hearing loss may be causing you. Answer YES, SOMETIMES, or NO for each question. To obtain a total score, add up the "yes" (4 points each), "sometimes" (2 points each), and "no" (0 points) responses. If your score is greater than 10, a hearing test is recommended.

Yes	Sometimes	No
4	2	0

E1 Does a hearing problem cause you to feel embarrassed when you meet new people?

E2 Does a hearing problem cause you to feel frustrated when talking to members of your family?

S1 Do you have difficulty hearing/understanding co-workers, clients, customers?

E3 Do you feel handicapped by a hearing problem?

S2 Does a hearing problem cause you difficulty when visiting friends, relatives or neighbors?

S3 Does a hearing problem cause you difficulty in the movies or in the theater?

E4 Does a hearing problem cause you to have arguments with family members?

S4 Does a hearing problem cause you difficulty when listening to TV or radio?

E5 Do you feel that any difficulty with your hearing limits or hampers your personal or social life?

S5 Does a hearing problem cause you difficulty when in a restaurant with relatives or friends?

Candidacy for Hearing Aids

We now know that your desire to purchase hearing aids is directly linked to a number of personal factors. These include:
1. your score obtained on the HHIE-S, HHIA-S, HHIE-SP;
2. your readiness for change;
3. and your motivational level

Bess[1] and his colleagues from Tennessee found that the extent of self-perceived hearing handicap on the 10-item screening version of the HHIE-S is predictive of hearing aid candidacy, in that it reliably distinguishes between people who ultimately purchase hearing aids and those who don't. Irrespective of the severity of hearing loss for pure tone signals (e.g. mild or moderate sensorineural hearing loss), persons in their study who actually purchased hearing aids were more handicapped as evidenced by higher scores on the HHIE-S, than those who did not.

Thus, the investigators concluded that when people perceive that a given hearing loss for pure tone signals is interfering with participation in and enjoyment of various activities, they are motivated to purchase hearing aids to reduce some of their communication difficulties.

Similarly, a study reported by Kochkin,[2] who sampled many hearing aid owners and non-owners across the country (presented in the previous chapter), revealed that an individual's total score on one of the hearing handicap inventories (HHI) statistically predicted ownership of hearing aids. For example, 5.7 percent of survey respondents who scored a "0" on the HHI owned a hearing aid whereas 49 percent of those with a score of "28" owned hearing aids. In general, this study revealed that the average score on the HHI of non-hearing aid owners was 13.7 out of a total score of 40, compared to 20.8 percent for hearing aid owners.

Interestingly, purchase of completely-in-the-canal (CIC) hearing aids is highly correlated to scores on the HHI as well. These studies demonstrate that self-perceived handicap, identified using a simple and easy screening tool, is linked to the decision on the part of individuals with hearing loss to purchase hearing aids. I encourage you to screen for the self-perceived effects of your loss using your hearing using one of the questionnaires included as Table 5-I or 5-II. If your total score adds up to 10 or more, you should schedule a hearing test and learn about the options available so that you don't have to miss out on hearing.

Clinically, I find that the sooner people come in for a hearing test, the more receptive they are to purchasing devices which may help overcome situation-specific difficulties such as understanding people on television or speech in large listening areas. Positive experiences with hearing assistive technologies, such as devices used with television or in theatres, often serve as an impetus to trying hearing aids.

The Impact of Hearing Loss

I would like to further elucidate on Dr. Kochkin's previous chapter with respect to how hearing loss can impact your quality of life with respect to benefitting from self-assessment qustionnaires. As you know by now, hearing loss restricts one or more dimensions in the quality of life including communication function, mental status, emotional and social function. Specifically, hearing impairment has been shown to:

- negatively impact on communicative behavior
- alter psychosocial behavior
- strain relations with friends or family members
- limit the enjoyment of daily activities
- jeopardize physical well-being
- interfere with the ability to live independently and safely
- potentially interfere with long distance contacts on the telephone
- compromise efficiency at work
- interfere with one's ability to work with co-workers, and clients
- interfere with medical diagnosis, treatment and management
- interfere with compliance with pharmacological regimens
- and interfere with therapeutic interventions across all disciplines including social work, speech-language therapy, physical or occupational therapy.

An interesting aspect of hearing impairment that afflicts adults is the large variability in response to a given hearing loss. That is to say, as stated elsewhere in this book, two individuals with the same amount of hearing loss can react very differently and can experience different behavioral consequences. Accordingly, more and more clinicians include as part of a complete hearing assessment, questions about how a given hearing loss impacts on communication, social and emotional function. The advent of digital signal processing and dual (directional) microphone technology, has revolutionized hearing aids to allow for enhanced listening comfort and optimal speech understanding in noise, and other difficult listening situations.

Data from a large scale study completed by the National Council on Aging[3] revealed objective evidence that hearing aids enable you to experience the personal stability and emotional fulfillment associated with interpersonal contacts and participation in everyday activities. Further, using change in responses to the HHI, clinicians have been able to document that hearing aids do in fact improve function in various social and emotional situations. We now know that the more hours per day one wears hearing aids, the greater the reduction in scores on the HHI—that is, the greater the improvement in social and emotional function.

Maximizing Benefit from Questionnaires

In 1996[4] and again in 2000,[5] I did a comprehensive review of studies on hearing aid benefit and satisfaction. It showed that hearing aids, either alone or in combination with three to six weeks of counseling-oriented audiological rehabilitation, do effectively reduce or minimize the disabilities and handicaps perceived by persons with adult onset sensorineural hearing loss. Further, they are a cost effective intervention for handicapping hearing loss and declining health associated with hearing loss.

More specifically, in approximately four to five studies conducted across the country in a number of different settings including private practices, hospital clinics, and veterans administration centers, 70 to 80 percent of new hearing aid wearers experienced very dramatic reductions in the amount of their self-perceived hearing handicap. That is to say, for example, hearing impairments which were initially judged to be moderately to severely handicapping (60 percent on the HHI) improved to the point that new hearing aid wearers considered their hearing loss to be slightly or mildly handicapping (20 percent on the HHI) after only three weeks of hearing aid use.

When these new hearing aid wearers were recalled to the hearing clinics to ascertain how they were functioning with their hearing aids, in many of the studies, they derived significant benefit such that they perceived the hearing loss to be less handicapping socially and emotionally. This is depicted in Figure 5-1 that shows a graph of how percentage handicap, as judged by clients according to their responses to the HHI, changed (improved) from 60 percent before hearing aids were purchased to 20 percent after three weeks and also after one year of hearing aid use.

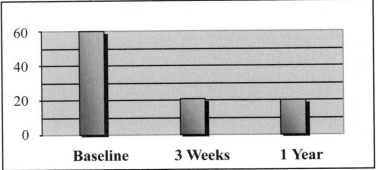

Figure 5-1: Improvement (reduction) in psychosocial handicap according to scores on the 25-item HHI following one-year of hearing aid use.

This represents a dramatic improvement and suggests that many of the problems people had when they came in for hearing aids—such as difficulty understanding friends, relatives, television and radio, or feeling upset by the hearing loss—were alleviated by hearing aid use. It is noteworthy that hearing aids did not "cure" each person's handicap.

The reality of hearing aids is that they're helpful in a variety of situations, and can alleviate feelings of isolation. However, it's unrealistic to expect "a quick fix" in all situations. Residual problems remain for which solutions are available as long as your hearing care practitioner has an open line of communication with you. Further, your expectations must be realistic so that you're not disappointed with hearing aid performance. A satisfied hearing aid wearer is one whose expectations match actual hearing aid performance.

There are times when new hearing aid wearers find they're not deriving the emotional and social benefits from hearing aids. For example, take the case of a 55-year-old teacher who recently found out that he had a mild to moderate sensorineural hearing loss. He had reported some difficulty understanding speech, especially in a noisy classroom. His score on the Hearing Handicap Inventory

(HHI) was 50 percent, suggesting that in fact he perceived his hearing loss as measured on the audiogram to be handicapping socially, emotionally and vocationally.

More particularly, he reported feeling handicapped, upset, embarrassed by and nervous from his inability to hear in a variety of situations, most notably at work (i.e. in the classroom), in movie theaters, and when socializing with friends and relatives. In light of his expenses at the time of the fitting, he decided to purchase binaural canal analog hearing aids. When he returned to his provider for the three-week follow-up appointment to determine how he was functioning with his hearing aids, he indicated that they were not helpful in the situations that mattered.

Further, he was annoyed by the sound of his voice with the hearing aids in his ears, and he noted that he heard whistling sounds a lot (feedback). His score on the long version of the HHI (i.e. 25 items) verified that the hearing aids, in fact, were not helping him, as the score remained at 50 percent, suggesting absolutely no benefit.

The hearing care professional suggested that the client try the newest technology—namely digital hearing aids with a dual microphone array and feedback controls. These units came with special earmolds that would help to make his voice sound more natural and the aids were equipped with special feedback elimination circuitry. He agreed to try them, was instructed on how to use them, was counseled regarding expected benefits, and returned one week later to pick up the hearing aids.

Three weeks later he returned for the follow-up visit. The client was quite pleased with the hearing aids, indicating that they were helpful in situations that were important to him and were alleviating some of the negative emotions attributable to his hearing loss. The aids felt more comfortable in his ear and he was not bothered by the quality of his voice or by annoying feedback. Above all, he felt less handicapped, anxious, and upset.

Responses to the HHI confirmed the client's subjective reports as his total score on the HHI improved to 10 percent suggesting a minimal hearing handicap with his new hearing aids. He continued to receive benefit after six months of hearing aid use. The pattern of findings is depicted in Figure 5-2. This case highlights the value of feedback from you, the client, and the importance of objectively quantifying performance with given hearing aids. Responses to a questionnaire, such as the HHI, can assist you in recognizing if and in what situations hearing aids are helping.

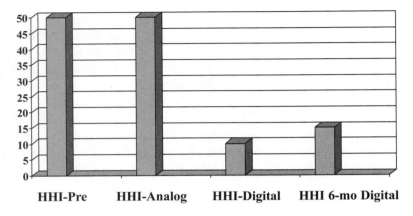

Figure 5-2: Score on the 25 item HHI with analog hearing aids (3 weeks post fitting), digital directional hearing aids (at 3 weeks and 6 months post fitting).

Another interesting way in which responses to the HHI can be helpful to both the new hearing aid wearer and the provider is when hearing aids seem helpful but their value does not seem to justify the expense. A retired attorney noted that now that he was no longer confined to an office or a courtroom, he was having difficulty functioning in the variety of new situations in which he found himself. He participated in a hearing screening at a local health fair and found out he was unable to hear pure tones being presented and scored an 18 on the screening version of the Hearing Handicap Inventory.

The clinician provided a referral to a hearing healthcare professional who urged him to obtain a complete hearing test. He scheduled an appointment with a provider and underwent a series of pure tone and speech tests to determine the extent of hearing loss. Results revealed a mild to moderate high frequency sensorineural hearing loss in each ear, consistent with the type of hearing loss attributable to the aging process. The score on the 25-item Hearing Handicap Inventory suggested a moderate psychosocial handicap (score of 40 percent).

In light of the client's complaints, the configuration of hearing loss (high frequency), and its severity (mild to moderate), binaural completely-in-the-canal hearing aids were recommended. The client was instructed to return to the provider after three weeks of hearing aid use to verify the response and monitor his performance with them.

Interestingly, on the return visit the client complained that the hearing aids were amplifying too much noise, and were not helpful in situations he considered most important (namely small groups) where background noise was present. The HHI score of 38 percent verified that in fact the hearing aids were not providing him with much assistance. After slight modification to the hearing aid response, the client left expressing satisfaction.

Upon the return visit (three weeks later, six weeks from the initial fitting), the client reported that the hearing aids were helping him to function well and enjoy numerous leisure activities in which he was participating. The HHI score at this time improved some 30 points to 8 percent, suggesting a minimal psychosocial handicap attributable to the hearing loss. Once again, objective verification for the client was helpful, enabling him to justify the expenditure.

There are occasions when individuals who were previously functioning well with their hearing aids can experience a decline in performance. Take for example the case of Mr. Osborn, an 80-year-old accountant who continues to work part-time. He had worn behind-the-ear hearing aids for 10 years and up until recently was quite satisfied with them. They were helping to alleviate his difficulties understanding speech, attributable to his bilateral, moderate, sensorineural hearing loss, which he first noted on his 65th birthday. Pure tone test results at his most recent examination by his provider revealed that his hearing loss had remained the same (moderate in degree).

However, his problems understanding speech had declined dramatically, especially in noisy situations. A complete audiological work-up revealed the possibility of an auditory processing problem. Noteworthy is the pattern of findings on the HHI confirmed Mr. Osborn's subjective complaints in that he no longer was benefiting from the hearing aids. As is evident from Figure 5-3, the initial HHI score was 50 percent (prior to hearing aids), improving to 24 percent after the initial hearing aid fitting. His HHI score was between 24 percent and 30 percent over time, suggesting considerable reduction (improvement) in psychosocial handicap attributable to hearing aid use.

Four years later, at Mr. Osborn's most recent visit, the HHI score returned to 52 percent, confirming limited hearing aid benefit. His provider recommended a conventional behind-the-ear aid with

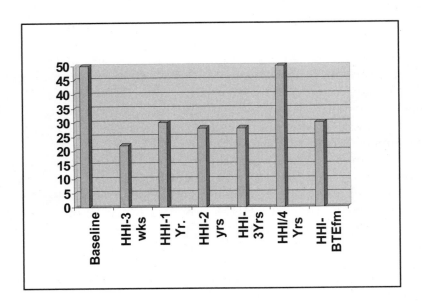

Figure 5-3: HHI scores over five-year time period with hearing aid and BTE/FM device.

an FM receiver incorporated into the hearing aid case. The advantage of an FM system is the improved signal-to-noise ratio achieved by bringing the microphone closer to the source of sound. Essentially, FM systems bridge the acoustical space between the sound source and the listener by eliminating the detrimental effects on speech understanding: distance, noise and reverberation.

The primary advantages of a BTE/FM system are that it can be used as a regular hearing aid, or as an FM receiver bringing the signal directly to the user's ear, or as both an FM system and a hearing aid. It's ideal when driving in a car, when conversing in a noisy environment, and when at a lecture or in a restaurant.

Mr. Osborn, at the urging of his wife, agreed to give the BTE/FM system a try and was immediately impressed with the clarity of the signal, especially when he was tested with noise present in the background. Mr. and Mrs. Osborn were counseled on how to use the hearing aids and upon their return visit were happy to report that speech understanding in the most difficult situations had improved dramatically. The HHI score of 28 percent verified that Mr. Osborn was deriving substantial benefit from the new device. Figure 5-3 summarizes the pattern of HHI scores over time with the hearing aids and with the BTE/FM system.

As hearing technology evolves and prices continue to rise, it is incumbent upon you to obtain information that can help you determine the value of hearing aids. Many hearing care practitioners have a variety of questionnaires at their disposal that can help you better understand how you function with hearing aids. This type of information can help to justify the high cost of present-day hearing aids. It is clear that hearing aids do provide quality of life benefits. Communication needs and expectations can be realized when hearing care professionals listen to you the consumer, either by modifying the response of a hearing aid, substituting one style hearing aid for another, or replacing a conventional hearing aid with some form of hearing assistive technology to ensure adequate benefit.

A Final Word

To gain full benefit from hearing aids, you must be informed, have realistic expectations and patience, and you must purchase hearing aids from a professional with whom you have confidence and rapport. It is also of utmost importance to have a firm idea about what you want from hearing aids. These are your self-perceptions.

Completion of a self-report questionnaire prior to and after purchasing hearing aids can help match perceptions of what you want hearing aids to do for you, against expectations as established by your hearing healthcare professional. The closer this match, the more satisfied you will be with hearing aids. Consider the self-report questionnaire as a checklist against which to judge the extent your needs are being met.

References

1. Bess F. Applications of the hearing handicap inventory for the elderly—screening version (HHIE-S). The Hearing Journal 48, 51-57, 1995.
2. Kochkin, S. MarkeTrak IV: 10-year trends in the hearing aid market-has anything changed? The Hearing Journal 49, 23-33, 1996.
3. National Council on the Aging. Report on the impact of untreated hearing loss in older Americans. Seniors Research Group, 1999.
4 Weinstein, B. Treatment efficacy: hearing aids in the management of hearing loss in adults. Journal Speech and Hearing Research 39,

S37-S45, 1996.

5. Weinstein, B. *Geriatric Audiology.* New York: Thieme Medical Publishers, Inc., 2000.

CHAPTER SIX
Hearing Aid Technology
Robert W. Sweetow, Ph.D.

Dr. Sweetow is Director of Audiology and Clinical Professor in the Department of
Otolaryngology at the Medical Center of the University of California, San Francisco.
He received his Ph.D. from Northwestern University in 1977. He holds a Master
of Arts degree from the University of Southern California and a Bachelor of Science
degree from the University of Iowa. Dr. Sweetow has lectured worldwide, and has
authored 20 textbook chapters and over 80 scientific articles on counseling, tinnitus
and amplification for the hearing impaired.

There are many myths and misconceptions regarding hearing
aids. The objective of this chapter is to prepare you with accurate
up-to-date information to help in your decision to upgrade or try new
hearing aids. As technology advances, and as social and workplace
demands change, so do the criteria for candidacy for wearable
amplification. Thirty-five years ago, many hearing healthcare
professionals believed that only people with conductive hearing loss
could be helped by hearing aids. Patients were often told that hearing
aids could make sounds *louder* (like turning up the volume on a radio),
but would not necessarily make sounds *clearer*. This thinking was
reinforced by reports of unfavorable results from those hearing
impaired patients who did try hearing aids and who still couldn't
understand speech clearly—particularly in noisy places.

Of course, it's now recognized that early attempts to fit
hearing aids on people with sensorineural loss were seriously hindered
by the limited sound quality produced by these early devices; by the
limited choice of electronic variations; and by poor fitting strategies
used in trying to determine the best manner to amplify speech without
making it too loud or too noisy.

In the early days of fitting hearing aids, professionals often
tried to determine who was a candidate on the basis of the degree of
hearing loss shown on the hearing test. You may recall that when
your hearing was tested, the audiologist or hearing instrument
specialist used beeping tones and made the sounds louder and softer
until you could no longer hear them. This very softest point, the point
at which you could just barely hear a sound is called your threshold.
These sounds are measured in decibels (dB). Classifications used two

decades ago stated that hearing better than 25 dB was normal; 26-50 dB was a mild loss; 51-70 dB was a moderate loss; 71-90 dB was a severe loss; and 91 dB and poorer was a profound loss. Strict application of these categories isn't adequate to describe the impact hearing loss has on your life. Indeed, it oversimplifies the complexities of hearing impairment. Today, we realize that *properly fitted hearing aids can provide benefit even if you have a relatively mild hearing loss.*

In addition to the previous belief among physicians and some hearing professionals that you couldn't successfully use hearing aids if you had nerve damage, it was also thought that you couldn't use hearing aids if you had normal hearing for low-pitched sounds (up to 1500 or 2000 Hz); or if you had a hearing loss in only one ear, or if your speech understanding abilities were reduced, and/or if you had difficulty tolerating loud sounds (for example, a crying baby). Advances in technology now allow for good fittings for most of these patients.

Present-Day Candidacy For Hearing Aids

In the past several years, hearing aid technology has advanced to the point where the question of candidacy is now based more on your communicative *needs* rather than purely on the test results obtained in a soundproof room. That is, your own personal, *subjective needs*. A good litmus test is to ask yourself whether you feel stressed or fatigued after a day of straining to hear. Hearing aids may simply relieve this strain, rather than making sounds louder or allowing you to understand all speech in all listening environments. Reducing strain alone can be a very significant benefit, not only to you, but to those trying to talk to you.

Occupational and social demands vary greatly among individuals. A judge who has a mild hearing loss may desperately need amplification, while a retired person living alone with the exact same degree of hearing loss may not. You must unselfishly examine whether you're becoming a burden to others, even if you do not personally recognize difficulty hearing. *Remember that wearing hearing aids may be a symbol of courtesy to others.* Unfortunately, despite the need, you, like many people, may resist trying hearing aids. Two common factors characterizing the response in people who have been told they should wear amplification are that practically no one wants to wear hearing aids, and no one wants to spend money or waste time solving a problem unless they perceive that a problem exists and a solution is readily attainable. Opposition to wearing hearing aids usually stems from three main reasons.

First is *hearsay*. Most everyone has friends or relatives who have purchased hearing aids currently residing in their dresser drawers. These unsuccessful wearers of amplification are more than happy to spread the gospel on the limitations (some accurate, some not) of hearing aids. Often, unsuccessful experiences occurred in extremely difficult listening environments in which even people with normal hearing had trouble understanding speech.

Second, despite the fact that people of all ages have hearing impairment and use amplification, there's an undeniable *social stigma* attached to wearing hearing aids. However, this problem has been eased by a continuing trend toward miniaturization of hearing aids, although not all listeners with hearing loss are candidates for tiny hearing aids. Stigma has also been greatly diminished by today's widespread use of wireless communications appliances.

The third main reason for opposition to hearing aid use is the perception that the relatively high cost of hearing aids is not reflected in the value and benefits they provide. When making a decision as to whether this is the right time for you to try hearing aids, you must weigh whether the financial investment can be offset by the improvement in your quality of life by reducing your hearing difficulty. Be sure to consider improvements from a social, emotional, and occupational perspective, also considering activities you would like to undertake but have given up because of communication difficulties.

It's a double-edged sword when it comes to dispensing hearing aids to a person who's not motivated to wear amplification. On one hand, a poorly motivated person is not the best candidate for amplification regardless of the degree of hearing loss. So, from this perspective, the answer to the question of whether a steadfastly reluctant patient should be forced into trying a hearing aid is probably *no*. It may be difficult to undo the damage that may be done if the borderline candidate prematurely tries, and fails with amplification. If you're absolutely opposed to trying hearing aids at this time, and if you're convinced you'll fail, it may be advisable to wait until another time when you may be more optimistic about the outcome.

On the other hand, keep in mind that it's very possible you will be pleasantly surprised. Remember that, as discussed later in this chapter, there have been more changes in hearing aids during the last few years than in the previous thirty.

Hearing Aid Styles

In the early 1950s, you would have been limited to a choice of two styles of hearing instruments: body borne or in-eyeglass frames. These devices are rarely seen today. However, you do have options regarding hearing aid styles (see: Figure 6-1). Behind-the-ear (BTE) hearing aids sit over the outer ear and are connected to an earmold located in the concha (bowl) of the ear and ear canal. There are a variety of sizes, shapes, and models of hearing aids that fit within a soft or hard plastic shell and are worn entirely inside the ear. They include the custom in-the-ear (ITE) model (which may completely fill, or occlude, the bowl and ear canal), the thinner low profile, the partially occluding half concha, the even less occluding helix model for high frequency losses, the in-the-canal (ITC), and the tiniest of styles, the completely-in-canal (CIC) hearing aids.

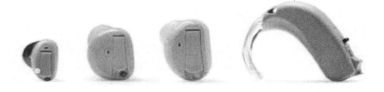

Figure 6-1: Range of hearing aid styles from (left to right) completely-in-the-canal to behind-the-ear.

I strongly discourage you from selecting the style of hearing aids you're going to try strictly on the basis of cosmetic factors. While cosmetic considerations may be important, the decision as to which style hearing aids are most appropriate for you should be based on both physical as well as audiological factors.

Physical factors

Anatomical characteristics may dictate the style; for example, behind-the-ear hearing aids may not be able to be used if you have deformed outer ears; the depth of your concha may determine the appropriateness of certain in-the-ear (ITE) model instruments; and in order to be able to wear the in-the-canal or the completely-in-canal types of hearing aids, your ear canal must be of sufficient diameter and must have a sharp enough bend to retain the aid, but not be so curvy that it prevents easy insertion and removal.

Manual dexterity is essential to handling some of the smaller style hearing aids. Not only is removal and insertion of canal hearing aids difficult for certain people, particularly as we get older, but the ability to manipulate any controls and the battery must be considered and assessed before you decide that a certain style is right for you. Also, some people need hearing aids that are large enough to accommodate a vent (hole) drilled into it, allowing air to enter the ear canal.

Without this ventilation, you may perceive a "plugged up" feeling or you may sound to yourself that you're "in a barrel" when you speak. This phenomenon is technically called the "occlusion effect." Some newer models of digital hearing aids greatly minimize the occlusion effect by allowing for more open ear fittings. In addition, if your ears produce excessive cerumen (earwax), you may be better off by not wearing canal, or even certain full ITE hearing aids.

Medical Contraindications such as draining ears or other medical problems may prevent the use of any hearing aid apparatus blocking your ear canals (see Chapter 8 Q&A #7 for complete medical contraindications). In this instance, you'll need open, non-occluding earmolds or possibly bone conduction-type systems. These types of hearing aids are beyond the scope of this discussion, and can be reviewed by your hearing healthcare provider if applicable to you.

Audiological factors:

The audiometric pattern on your audiogram may show certain frequencies (pitches) that have normal hearing. For example, in the low frequencies, you may be best served by systems that don't occlude (block) your ear canal and thus allow low-pitched sounds to pass into your ear without being amplified.

The degree of loss may predict the need for a specific kind of hearing aid. For example, severe and profound hearing losses are best served by BTE-style hearing aids.

Special features may be indicated, such as directional or multiple microphones (which primarily amplify signals coming from in front of you) and/or the addition of a telecoil (a magnetic induction loop). Telecoils allow sound to bypass the hearing aid microphone and amplify signals received electromagnetically (from telephones). In addition to allowing a hearing aid wearer to listen to telephone signals without getting feedback (whistling), telecoils can interface with a variety of assistive listening devices (see Appendix I).

Acoustic feedback refers to the whistling or ringing sound often produced when you cup your hand or a telephone over your ear while wearing a hearing aid. It also occurs when the hearing aid or earmold is not properly or snugly inserted in your ear. Before discussing feedback, it would help to first describe the basic components of hearing aids.

Figure 6-2 shows the series of events that occur in conventional, non-digital hearing aids: First, sound enters into a microphone. Next, this sound is transformed into an electrical current as the diaphragm of the microphone moves back and forth. Then, the electrical current is fed into an amplifier and filtered by electrical components that establish how much relative amplification will be provided for the different frequencies. For example, most hearing aids try to amplify the high pitches more than the low pitches. The overall amount of amplification may be governed by a volume control . The newly formed amplified electrical signal is then fed to a receiver, also called a loudspeaker. The receiver turns the electrical signal back into sound waves that exit the hearing aid and enter the ear canal through the earmold for BTE hearing aids, or a tube in the plastic shell for custom styles.

Also, all hearing aids are run by a tiny battery, which generally lasts for between one to three weeks. The basic design of digital hearing aids, that will be discussed later in this chapter, differ in that they contain a signal processor rather than an amplifier and they often adjust the volume automatically without the need for volume controls.

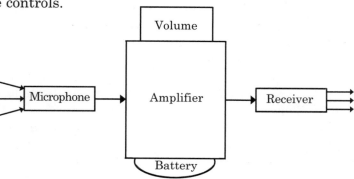

Figure 6-2: Transmission of sound through a hearing aid.

Generally speaking, the closer the microphone is to the exit point of the amplified sound from the hearing aid or earmold, the greater the likelihood of feedback. Feedback occurs when amplified sound from the earmold leaks back into the hearing aid's microphone and is re-amplified. This is a very important consideration in the selection and fitting of amplification. BTE hearing aids often have an advantage over smaller ITE or ITC styles in this regard since there's more physical distance between the microphone and the receiver.

Conventional hearing aids provide "feedback controls" which are adjustments that reduce high frequency amplification. While this does indeed accomplish the desired effect of reducing feedback, it may do so at the expense of also reducing the audibility of the vitally important high frequency consonant sounds that are essential for understanding speech. Therefore, this approach to feedback control is often not an acceptable compromise. The newest generation of advanced digital hearing aids has "active feedback management" systems. An active system detects feedback and counteracts it before it occurs by sending out counter signals to cancel the feedback.

In any case, it's important that the earmolds or hearing aid shells fit perfectly in your ears. This is why it's essential that your hearing healthcare professional takes good impressions of your ears before you obtain hearing aids. If you haven't yet had an earmold impression taken, don't worry. It doesn't hurt. Your provider will first place a cotton or foam block in your ear canal and will then inject liquid material in your ear that will harden in about five minutes. It's a similar process to getting impressions made by the dentist, except thankfully, you don't need the Novocain shot!

Small Hearing Aids

If you're like most patients, perhaps one of the first questions you have is whether you can use one of the really small, "invisible" hearing aids (the ITC or CIC styles). Hearing aids keep getting smaller but small does not necessarily mean better. A canal-style hearing aid implies that no part of the hearing aid extends into the concha (bowl) area. There are two types: the ITC aid fills the outer half, or soft, cartilaginous portion of the ear canal while the CIC is inserted deeper in the ear canal and extends into the inner half. The CIC hearing aid is so tiny that it must be removed from the ear by pulling on a removal wire that rests at the bottom of the concha.

Advantages Of CIC Hearing Aids:

- They are the most *"invisible"* systems available.
- The microphone lies either within, or at the entrance of the ear canal and thus is able to benefit fully from the *natural amplification* of the outer ear bowl.
- The receiver of the hearing aid is located closer to the eardrum, where the amount of air trapped in the ear canal that needs to vibrate is less than for most other fittings. Therefore, *less hearing aid amplification is needed* to produce the same sound pressure at the eardrum. This often results in lower distortion levels and less likelihood of acoustic feedback.

Disadvantages of CIC Hearing Aids:

- If the receiver stops in the outer half of the canal, it may be *subject to breakdowns* due to blockage from earwax.
- With certain basic instruments, if the receiver terminates in the outer cartilaginous portion of the canal, you may notice the "occlusion" or "barrel effect" in which your *own voice sounds hollow* as if you were in a tunnel. Digital technology can help reduce or even eliminate this effect.
- If the receiver stops in the inner, bony portion of the canal, this deeper canal placement may be *physically uncomfortable* to you because the skin is much thinner than it is at the outer part of the canal.
- Because the aid is so small, *there may not be enough space to vent the aid* in order to relieve pressure build-up, release unwanted low frequency amplification, or to house multiple microphones or telecoils.
- They are *not powerful enough to fit severe or profound losses.*
- Adequate manual *dexterity for changing the tiny batteries is essential.*

It's not unusual to find that the most important factors determining success or failure of a fitting are those unrelated to audiometric findings. In particular, you must take into consideration all of the following: your age and general physical and mental health; your motivation (as opposed to that of your family's); finances; cosmetic considerations; and your communication needs. It's heartening to note that the primary reasons for rejection of hearing aids, after people try them, are less related to finances and cosmetics, and more to do with difficulty hearing in background noise, and discomfort from loud sounds. These problems are well on the way to being lessened by modern-day hearing aids and fitting techniques.

The Evolution of Hearing Aids

There are three basic rules that must be followed if a hearing aid fitting is to be successful: soft sounds must be made audible; normal conversational sounds must be comfortable; and loud sounds must not be uncomfortable. The reason is that if you have a sensorineural hearing loss, your hearing loss is for soft sounds but not for loud sounds. Therefore, hearing aids have changed over the past three decades in the following ways.

1. Linear Hearing Aids

In the past, many wearers reported that in order to hear soft sounds, they had to turn their hearing aids up quite high. This did indeed allow them to hear soft sounds but it also produced the undesirable effect of making loud sounds uncomfortable. Here's why.

Imagine that a certain level of sound enters the hearing aid, let's say 65 dB (which happens to be about the level of normal conversational speech). To make this speech comfortable, the volume of the hearing aid might be set so that it produces 25 dB of amplification. Therefore, 90 dB comes into the ear canal (65 plus 25).

Now, lets imagine that the sound coming into the hearing aid suddenly becomes much louder, as might occur in a restaurant when people at your table start to laugh at a joke. If you are wearing a linear hearing aid, the sound coming into it is now increased to 80 dB, and this type of hearing aid will still add 25 dB of amplification, so the sound in your ear canal actually becomes 105 dB. For most people, this will be entirely too loud and uncomfortable, and your reaction will be to try and turn it down using the volume control. This is why you'll see most people with linear hearing aids turning the volume control quite often when the sound intensity in the surrounding environment changes. Hearing aids which produce the same amount of amplification regardless of the loudness of the sound entering are technically categorized as *linear, one channel, conventional* hearing aids.

2. Non-Linear, *Single Channel*

In 1992, a new type of hearing aid was introduced using more advanced technology called non-linear, or dynamic range compression. With this system, there's more amplification given to soft sounds than there is for louder sounds. In other words, when sounds are above a certain level set in the hearing aid, it's as if an invisible finger reaches up and automatically moves the volume down for you, and vice versa, when the sound environment becomes lower than a certain level it moves the volume up for you.

This type of non-linear hearing aid basically squeezes a wide range of loudness into a narrower range, which has generated the other descriptive name of *compression hearing aids*. Going back to the earlier example, now with the non-linear type, when sounds entering the hearing aid suddenly increase to 80 dB, the amplification may be lowered from 25 dB to 10 dB. Therefore, the sound reaching your eardrum is a more comfortable 90 dB as opposed to the uncomfortable 105.

3. Non-Linear, *Multichannel*

While non-linear, single channel hearing aids help maintain comfortable loudness perception, another limitation remains: Your loudness growth pattern may be different from one pitch to another. That is, you might find that high-pitched sounds (like dishes clanging) seem painfully loud to you but low-pitched sounds (a refrigerator humming) do not. Therefore, the amount of compression may need to be different for various frequencies. This is where the next step up in circuitry sophistication comes in, *non-linear multiple channel*.

With multiple channels, compression characteristics of the hearing aid will be tailored to your personal needs based upon how loud you interpret certain sounds to be for various frequencies. Perhaps there will be a lot of compression for the high frequencies but very little for the low frequencies. Compression helps to make sounds appear comfortably loud for you.

The second thing multichannel compression accomplishes may be even more important. If your hearing aid system has only one channel, a loud noise made up of mostly low frequencies (as might be found in cocktail parties) would instruct the hearing aid that it needs to lower its amplification for all frequencies. This would help to keep the sound from being too loud, but it would make some of the high frequency sounds (like consonants) too soft to hear.

On the other hand, a multichannel hearing aid, in that same loud, low frequency noise situation, would decrease the amplification for low frequencies, making sound comfortable without changing the amplification for the high frequencies (thus preserving audibility of important high frequency consonant sounds). This system can actually produce additional high frequency amplification while simultaneously reducing low frequency amplification, all depending on the sound environment.

Non-linear, multiple channel hearing aids act not only as a means of loudness control, but also as a means of differentiating the amount of amplification given to different parts of the speech signal. If fitted correctly, they can dampen the strong elements of speech, such as vowels, and enhance the delicate speech elements such as the /s/, /sh/ and /f/ sounds. This will greatly improve speech clarity, especially in difficult listening environments.

4. Multiple Programs versus Automatic

Some people find it useful to be able to change hearing aid characteristics depending on the environment they are in. Of course, you can't keep running back to your provider each time you enter a new environment. Another option would be to have hearing aids that have several programs that you can easily select simply by touching a button located on the hearing aid or on a separate remote control. For example, one button could select a hearing aid program which is best suited to listening to one person, another program to listening in a restaurant, and yet another for music. This can also be useful if you have a fluctuating hearing loss.

Many modern hearing aids are automatic in the way they regulate volume. Often, these hearing aids regulate themselves so automatically that they don't contain a volume control. You may find this to your liking if you're the type who doesn't like to frequently adjust your hearing aids, or, you may feel that not having a volume control takes away too much control from you. This is something you should discuss carefully with your hearing healthcare provider.

5. Digitally-Programmable Hearing Aids

Hearing aids that are programmed, or set, by your hearing healthcare provider, via an external computer, or computer-like instrument are called *digitally programmable*. This does not mean you own a "digital" hearing aid. It merely means the computer process for programming is digitally based. The basic advantage of programmable is the flexibility for your hearing care professional to change the characteristics in the hearing aids as your needs may change. Often, preferences for sound amplification changes over time after you have used the hearing aids for a while.

For instance, if you're a new wearer, you may not want hearing aids to amplify high pitches too much because they might seem too sharp or tinny. But after you've grown accustomed to hearing sounds you may not have heard for a long time, you may want to hear some of these high-pitched sounds. With a programmable system, your hearing healthcare provider can alter the amplification in your instruments by boosting higher pitches.

6. Directional and Multiple Microphone Hearing Aids

Typically, you face the person who is speaking to you. Noise, however, may originate in front, behind, and/or to your sides. Many programmable and digital hearing aids contain directional or multiple microphones that "communicate" with each other so that sounds originating from the front of the hearing aid receive maximum amplification, and sounds originating from the sides or behind receive less amplification. This effectively suppresses some of the annoying background noise that may create so much difficulty for you.

Some hearing aids allow you to select whether you want most of the amplification to occur for signals in front of you or whether you want equal amplification for signals all around you. An example of when you might want amplification to occur from all around you would be when listening to music. Other multiple microphone hearing aids make these adjustments automatically for you.

7. Digital Hearing Aids

The most advanced hearing aids today use fully digital processing. A digital hearing aid has a computer chip performing the amplification steps instead of the traditional analog circuitry. It's actually a miniature computer in itself. This is a major breakthrough in technology because it greatly increases the amount of sound processing possible in the given amount of space.

The improvement from digital hearing aids is exciting and far-reaching because they have minimal distortion, a clearer/crisper quality, advanced feedback control, improved noise suppression, and occlusion (hollow sound) management. The first commercially available digital hearing aids took all the benefits from the advanced non-linear multichannel hearing aids and improved them even further. They have the ability to analyze the sound environment and adapt the amplification accordingly, making speech clearer. This is all done automatically without the need for volume or remote controls.

Second generation digital hearing aids that recently were introduced have more "intelligence built into the chips," allowing them to recognize the difference between the human voice versus incoming noise, and further improve speech perception. Once third and fourth generation chips are developed, they will allow for even more processing capabilities.

Limitations Of Hearing Aids

Hearing aids are meant to minimize listening fatigue and to improve ease of communication. They're not meant to allow you to "hear a pin drop," and there are going to be circumstances in which hearing aids don't give you all the benefits you'd like. The most frequent complaints voiced by hearing aid wearers are that noise is amplified too much, certain sounds become too loud to bear, and some speech remains unclear.

No hearing aids effectively eliminate all background noise. If all the sound energy that makes up noise were eliminated, important segments of speech also would be missing. And, remember that normal listeners experience background noise daily. If all background noise were eliminated, the acoustic world would be quite boring and unnatural. Even so, don't hesitate to discuss your perception of background noise with your provider so that your hearing aids can be fine-tuned to reach the best compromise. Some of the newer digital instruments have automatic modes, decreasing fatigue and only boosting amplification when speech is present.

With regard to clarity, remember that hearing aids are *aids* to hearing. They are not new ears, and they cannot correct for certain limitations in understanding that are more related to brain functioning and poor listening habits than to hearing.

You may find that your own voice sounds odd when wearing

hearing aids. The reason this occurs is that when you speak, you produce low frequency vibrations in your ear canals. When you're unaided, your ears are open, allowing these vibrations to escape from your ear canals out into the air. As touched on earlier, if your ears are blocked, these low frequency sounds are trapped in your ear canals and cannot escape. This increase in low frequency perception might make you sound as if you were talking in a barrel or experiencing an echo.

This "occlusion effect" can be minimized by: 1) keeping the ear as open as possible, perhaps by means of vents (holes) drilled into the earmold or plastic shell; 2) reducing low frequency amplification; 3) using an earmold or ITE shell that sits deeply, reaching the inner half of the canal, thus reducing vibration; 4) or in some cases, having the canal portion of the shell not set rather shallow in the ear.

As mentioned earlier, a common annoyance with all but the latest generation digital hearing aids is the presence of feedback. Feedback doesn't mean that the hearing aid is malfunctioning. There are two types of acoustic feedback: that produced internally from the hearing aid indicating the need for repair, and the more common external feedback produced by leakage of amplified sound out of the ear canal and back into the microphone of the hearing aid. Usually, external feedback can be corrected by 1) re-positioning or possibly remaking the earmold or the plastic shell; 2) plugging, or reducing the diameter of any vents; or 3) reducing the amount of high frequency amplification, which is usually an unacceptable trade-off because of the resultant loss of high frequency consonant audibility.

Another common limitation of hearing aids is that you may have more difficulty hearing when the sound source is at a distance from you. This occurs, for example, in large conference rooms or auditoriums. Loudness (intensity) decreases as physical distance increases. Unfortunately, most background noise surrounds you, so while the intensity of speech decreases with distance, the intensity of noise may not. This is one reason why hearing aids effectively transmit sound if the speaker talks right into the microphone, but at longer, more realistic distances, reception diminishes. It would be ideal if sound produced at the source transferred directly to you without losing any intensity. It's obviously impractical, however, to ask someone speaking to you to constantly move closer to your ear.

One way to achieve this effect is with direct audio input, where the person speaking holds or wears a microphone. Unfortunately, many hearing aid wearers are reluctant to ask others to use a microphone or wear a wired device. An alternative approach is to use instruments called assistive listening devices that transmit by wireless FM (like a radio), infrared, or induction loop. You may have seen these devices in auditoriums and theaters, and they can be used in combination with your hearing aids.

Realistic Expectations With New Hearing Aids

As I mentioned earlier, hearing aids are not new ears; they are electronic devices; they are not perfect; and for the most part, they do not eliminate background noise. Since many patients with sensorineural hearing loss deny the presence of a hearing impairment, or lack sufficient motivation, they often demand to be convinced of the improvement that hearing aids might offer. Since the main goal of amplification is to facilitate the ease of communication, don't be disappointed if you experience only minimal benefit during the initial trial with amplification.

The benefit derived from amplification may be subtle. Depending on your hearing loss, the goal of the hearing aids may not be to make sounds louder. That is, especially where only high frequency amplification occurs, there are only a few English language sounds in this range (such as /s/, /sh/, /t/, /th/, /f/, and /k/). Therefore, your hearing aids are designed to pick up only these consonants and since we're talking about relatively few sounds, the benefits of amplification may not be readily apparent. It's important to note here that even though we're speaking of a few sounds, these sounds are critically important.

You also need to recognize that prediction of guaranteed long-term benefit from amplification is difficult to determine. A period of initial adjustment and a learning process is required for most new hearing aid users. It may take several weeks before you adjust to the new pattern of sound and learn new "recognition" cues that you probably have not heard for a long time. As a new wearer, you need to be oriented to the world of amplification. You may require a gradual "break-in" wearing schedule (a few hours the first day, six hours the second, nine hours the third, etc.), or you may be encouraged to wear the hearing aids immediately during all your waking hours. You may require additional counseling and training, either individually, or in groups with others with hearing loss, and family members.

You must accept that time is required for adapting to hearing aids. Your ability to understand amplified speech can continue to grow for as long as three months following the use of a new hearing aids.

Most hearing healthcare professionals will give you a one-month trial period with new hearing aids. If market conditions allow, trial periods may be extended. My advice is, if a trial period is not offered, take your business elsewhere!

It's important that you read the instruction manual that comes with your hearing aids. Hopefully, your provider will have told you everything you need to know about inserting and removing your hearing aids, checking the batteries, cleaning and maintaining the instruments, and using hearing aids with the telephone. But often, too much information can overload the brain! Take the hearing aids home, read the instruction manual, and then call your provider if you have any questions. Then go out and wear them in a variety of listening environments. When you return to your hearing healthcare provider, discuss the situations with which you may have had difficulty so that possible adjustments and fine-tuning can be achieved.

Also remember that hearing aids are sophisticated electronic devices that spend most of their time in a rather unfriendly environment—your ear. Can you imagine what would happen if you placed your home stereo system in a rainforest? Well, your ear canal is somewhat like a rainforest in that it is very warm (about 98.6 degrees), it's moist (with earwax), and it doesn't always receive enough fresh air. As such, hearing aids do require occasional repair. Blockage from earwax is the most common cause for hearing aid malfunction. Ask your hearing aid provider about some of the modern "wax traps" that can help keep earwax out of your hearing aids. You can minimize the need for repair if you are conscientious about cleaning them daily according to instructions and possibly storing them every night in a container that soaks up any excess moisture (see Chapter 9 on maintenance).

Conclusions

Now you have the facts, at least as they stand early in the 21st century. Remember, in order to have the best chance of succeeding with hearing aids, be patient with yourself and maintain realistic expectations. You and your brain have consciously and subconsciously created many behaviors to compensate for your hearing loss over the years. Some of the habits you have picked up have truly helped your ability to communicate, but some may have actually impaired your communication skills.

CHAPTER SEVEN
Why Some Consumers Reject Hearing Aids But How You Could Love Them!
Sergei Kochkin, Ph.D.

Dr. Kochkin is a Director of Market Development & Market Research at Knowles Electronics and past member of the Board of Directors of the Better Hearing Institute in Washington, D.C. He has published more than 50 papers on the hearing aid market and conducted customer satisfaction research on more than 25,000 hearing aid owners. He holds a Doctorate in psychology, an MBA in marketing, a Masters of Science in counseling and guidance and a BA in physical anthropology & archeology. Dr. Kochkin also maintains an interest in ancient cultures, comparative religion and meditation.

Recent research in the United States indicates that close to 29 million people have a hearing loss, or nearly one in ten Americans. In addition, about 1.2 million school-age children have a hearing loss. The early identification and treatment of hearing loss in children is particularly critical since hearing is synonymous with normal development of speech. It is important that you understand the prevalence of hearing loss, and that it cuts across all age groups. In focus groups with people who have rejected hearing aids, some people with hearing loss have come to the erroneous conclusion that they are a rare or obscure individual, "since so few people have hearing loss." When shown that they are not alone, they tend to be more accepting of their hearing loss and therefore more willing to seek out a hearing aid solution.

From conversations with experts in other countries, it's generally recognized that close to ten percent of the populations in developed countries have problems with their hearing. I happen to believe this figure may be higher, because most studies do not include hearing loss populations in institutional settings such as nursing or retirement homes, the military, and prisons. Among the elderly, hearing loss is the third most serious health issue, following arthritis and hypertension.

The vast majority *(close to 90-95 of people with hearing loss)* can be helped by hearing aids. There have been major breakthroughs in hearing aid technology in very recent years, and we can now do a better job of matching technology with a candidate's lifestyle and communication needs. Yet, some hearing aids still end up in a drawer.[1]

The good news is that many of the problems with hearing aids have been solved, and wearers can now expect improved communication with hearing aids as the rule, not the exception.

Why do some individuals have difficulty adjusting to hearing aids while others are doing so well that people around them don't even notice they're wearing them? What's different about successful hearing aid wearers? And why do only one in five individuals with hearing loss use hearing aids despite the proven value of amplification. Some interesting facts are now coming to light, which may answer these questions.

Why Some People Reject Hearing Aids

More than 22 million people in the United States have never tried hearing aids as a solution to their hearing loss. In one research investigation, close to 3,000 individuals with self-reported hearing loss were polled regarding their reluctance to try hearing aids.[2] Here are some of the reasons why consumers have declined to pursue them.

1. Inadequate information

Many people are not aware they have a significant hearing loss and therefore are in need of information that would help them recognize it. Most people lose hearing gradually. In most cases, it's slowly progressive. During this time, the person with hearing loss and family members learn to adapt to it, often not even realizing that they're doing this. The number one reason why people buy their very first hearing aid is the "recognition that their hearing got worse;" usually this means they made embarrassing mistakes in society due to their untreated hearing loss. Thus, one of the first things individuals with suspected hearing loss should do is determine if they exhibit some of the signs of hearing loss.

2. Stigma and Cosmetics

Some people reject hearing aids because they are concerned with the stigma of hearing loss or are in a state of denial, and thus try to hide it from others. It's unfortunate, but many people, because they have less than perfect hearing, believe they are inferior, unintelligent, or simply less lovable. They believe other people will think they're getting older or that they will be viewed as less competent, less attractive, and so on. They may have shame regarding their hearing loss. This is partly due to the fact that we live in a youth-oriented, airbrushed society where physical perfection is stressed as an important human attribute.

As you previously read in this book, cosmetics no longer need to be a barrier to obtaining amplification. Since the 1990s, technological advances have permitted the hearing aid industry to develop hearing instruments like the completely-in-the-canal (CIC) devices, which are essentially not very visible (see Figure 6-1, page 96). In fact, research shows that 90 percent of consumers perceive these CICs to be completely invisible. Based on your hearing needs and the physical characteristics of your ears, you might be a candidate for these "invisible devices." If you're not, rest assured that in-the-canal (ITC) devices, although larger, are available to fit many hearing losses and are not terribly noticeable.

Understand though, that once you begin hearing through amplification and once your quality of life is enhanced, cosmetics will be of lesser concern to you. Research shows that people who have come to enjoy their hearing aids rate even the largest hearing aids as cosmetically appealing as compared to some of the smaller, in-the-ear models.[3] Some hearing instruments even come in bright colors—dispelling the myth that they are something to be ashamed of or hide!

3. Misdirected Medical Guidance

Many people have received misinformation about their hearing loss from well-intending physicians, and the extent to which it can be helped. For instance, many physicians have recommended to their patients that they're not candidates for hearing aids if they have hearing loss in one ear and good hearing in the other *(unilateral hearing loss)*; if they have "nerve deafness" *(an obsolete term for sensorineural hearing loss)*; or if the hearing loss still allows them to conduct a conversation in quiet. Many times the doctor's opinion will be based on the fact that the patient and doctor are able to conduct a face-to-face conversation while in the secluded and usually quiet exam room. Much of this misinformation is given unintentionally by family physicians who do not specialize in hearing problems. In fact, most physicians (except ear, nose and throat specialists) receive very little training in medical school in the areas of hearing loss and hearing aids.

4. Not Realizing the Importance of Hearing

Another reason for rejection of hearing aids is that people have forgotten how important hearing is to their quality of life. We live in such a visually oriented society that often hearing plays a secondary role. As you know from your own experience, or from reading this book, people who cannot hear well, often have lives filled with anxiety, insecurity, isolation and depression. People gradually withdraw from family and friends because without auditory contact they lose the feeling of being connected. In essence, they grow numb to the world around them. But in the world, communication is critical. We interact with one another through communication.

I am aware of a CEO who lost more than a million dollars in business because he misunderstood a client's needs; learning from this mistake he always wears his hearing aids when meeting with clients especially when negotiating a contract. I am aware of a grandfather who was thought to be senile instead of hearing impaired. He was able to compensate for his hearing loss with hearing aids and began to effectively interact with his family again. Most hearing healthcare professionals know of horror stories of children being misdiagnosed as slow, retarded, hyperactive, or having poor attention spans when in fact it was impaired hearing.

5. Misbelief that Hearing Aids Don't Work

A significant number of people with hearing loss mistakenly believe that hearing aids are not effective for what they are designed to do. Many people judge hearing aids based on what they've seen their grandparents wear—a large, clunky box about the size of a pack of cigarettes with wires coming out of it.

Recent research with consumers utilizing a variety of hearing aids *(high technology as well as older technology aids 1-5 years old)* indicates that 76 percent of hearing aid wearers report satisfaction *(defined as satisfied or very satisfied)* with the ability of the hearing aid to improve their hearing, and 66 percent report that hearing aids have significantly improved the quality of their life.[4] If this research had been conducted twenty years ago, this high satisfaction factor probably would not have even been 35 percent. A significant number of people report satisfaction with their hearing aids in quiet situations (87 percent) as well as in very difficult situations such as restaurants, places of worship or large groups.

In research with more than 25,000 consumers I have learned

that not everyone benefits equally in all listening situations, nor do all types of hearing aid circuitry perform the same in difficult listening situations. As an example, the average hearing aid achieves a 30 percent satisfaction rating in noisy situations; yet some technologies, notably programmable hearing aids with multiple microphones *(known as directional hearing aids)*, achieve satisfaction ratings as high as 67 percent.[3] Similarly, only about 41 percent of consumers are satisfied with hearing aids on the telephone, yet, some instruments, such as completely-in-the-canal (CIC) hearing aids perform better on the phone as well as outdoors because they're located just inside the entrance of the ear canal and produce less feedback while on the phone. Much of this satisfaction may also be due to diminished wind noises outdoors, a sense of more natural amplification, and the need for somewhat less power resulting in increased tolerance while in the presence of background noise.

6. Failure to Trust in a Hearing Aid Dispensing Professional

Another key reason some people hold off their purchase is: "I do not trust hearing health providers who fit hearing aids!" The data show that nearly 90 percent of consumers are satisfied with their hearing aid dispensing professional.[4] It is certainly worth mentioning that the training, education and experience among dispensers of hearing aids has greatly increased over the years for both audiologists and hearing instrument specialists (see Chapter 2).

7. Unrecognized Value of Hearing Aids

Many people who have avoided amplification tend to believe there is little value in hearing aids. By low value they mistakenly assume that "hearing aids will not work for them" and therefore they will not derive any benefit. Both consumers and physicians have little knowledge of the potential benefit of hearing aids. Since the new millennium, large-scale research has been published on the impact of hearing aids on quality of life for people who use hearing aids in the United States.[5] While I have devoted a full chapter to this research, it is important that we summarize this impact here.

In my humble opinion, I cannot think of a consumer product with such an impressive list of potential benefits: greater earning power, improved interpersonal relationships, reduced discrimination toward the person with the hearing loss, reduced difficulty in communicating, less need to compensate for hearing loss, reduced anger and frustration, reduction in depression and anxiety, enhanced emotional stability, reductions in paranoid feelings, reduced social phobias, greater belief that you are in control of your life, reduced self-criticism, increased self-esteem, improved perceptions of mental acuity, improved health status, greater level of outgoingness (e.g. extroversion) and greater likelihood of participating in groups. I challenge anyone to name a product or a service with this impressive list of benefits. When I presented these findings to a group of medical doctors, one prominent physician stated, *"I was not aware of the seriousness of hearing loss and the potential for hearing aids to alleviate the problem. Every doctor in the world must be made aware of these findings!"*

8. Feeling Priced Out of the Market

Some people with hearing loss simply do not have the disposable income that would enable them to afford today's modern hearing aids. Based on the known benefits of hearing aids in improving quality of life there is some effort to see if more government programs such as Medicare will cover hearing aids. If the person with a hearing loss is a child many local and state governments offer hearing aids at no or reduced cost. Check to see if you qualify for free, or a reduced price for hearing aids through your union, employer, the Veterans Administration, your insurance provider, local HMO or your local Lions Club.

Ten Ways to Optimize your Chances of Being A Satisfied Hearing Aid Wearer

There is nothing more important to the manufacturers of hearing aids and hearing health professionals than your satisfaction with their product and services. Like any smart businessman, they know that satisfied consumers lead to repeat business and to positive word-of-mouth advertising for their products. The hearing aid industry is interested in delighting you, in meeting your needs and exceeding your expectations. The hearing aid industry is people-oriented in that it allows significant interaction and communication between the person with the hearing loss and the hearing health professional to assure that they have done all things possible to meet your needs. It is important to emphasize that you have a roll to play in assuring your satisfaction with hearing aids. So, I would like to offer some suggestions for optimizing the chances that you will be one of these delighted hearing aid wearers.

1. Meeting Your Needs

Simply stated, satisfaction is having your needs, desires or expectations met. Another way of looking at satisfaction is that you are fulfilled, based on a promise which may have come from the hearing care provider, literature, a website, advertising or a mixture of these sources. You have very specific needs and the purpose of the hearing health provider is to find out what your needs are and to meet them. Thus, during the process of rediscovering your hearing it is important to determine what your needs are, what outcomes you are looking for, and most importantly, how you'll know when you've fulfilled your needs. Many people go into their hearing health practitioner with a vague concept of their need: "I can't hear," or "It seems as if people are mumbling more," or worse yet, "My wife says I don't listen to her."

I believe you will have a more fulfilling hearing aid experience if you dig deeper to comprehend the impact your hearing loss has had on your life emotionally, behaviorally, mentally and socially. There are a number of chapters in this book that can help you in this task. Write the issues down because they will become a roadmap for both you and your hearing health professional. Also, many hearing health professionals have assessment scales that will help you understand problems caused by your hearing loss (as described in Chapter 5). Once you know your problems, you can better identify your expected outcomes. It's your personal needs list and when it's fulfilled it will bring a smile to your face and the faces of your loved ones. This list also becomes a contract between you and your hearing care professional.

Identification of communication situations that cause you the most difficulty is a critical first step in solving your hearing loss problems. If you can describe difficult listening conditions, your hearing care provider can address the problems and develop strategies to help you manage them. If you need more information, ask for it. Some people want highly technical information about hearing aid systems and hearing loss, while others just want a brief overview of hearing aids and their function. Most providers will be happy you asked, and will give you information such as consumer literature, data sheets, brochures, videotapes and other types of instructional materials. Ask for clarification if you need it. Many complex concepts can be explained in an uncomplicated way.

2. Motivation

Advanced hearing aid technology can now compensate for most hearing losses, but there are still millions of hearing aid candidates who are not ready to accept this fact. Is there a missing link? I think so. People with hearing loss are in different stages of readiness. At one extreme the individual is in denial about the hearing loss. If either a family member or a professional insists on hearing aids at this point, behavior is unlikely to change and most likely such a person would be dissatisfied if pursuing hearing aids.

Individuals highly motivated to improve their hearing have an infinitely better chance of success with hearing aids. Such motivated people recognize their hearing loss and are open to change. They tend to seek out relevant information related to their hearing loss and the technology needed to alleviate their hearing loss. The most highly motivated hearing aid candidates have a willingness to discuss their feelings about their hearing loss problem and explore some hearing options that might be available to them. When they are fitted with hearing aids, they eagerly explore their new technology, discuss problems during follow-up visits with their hearing health professional, and patiently learn to adapt to their technology.

3. Positive Attitude

The most important personality trait that one could possess is a positive attitude, not just toward the process of obtaining hearing aids, but toward life in general. Motivation is a key to success with amplification. This means a willingness to try hearing aids, adapt to new solutions, and keep frustration at a minimum when obstacles arise. If you view your circumstances as beyond your control, there's a higher probability that you'll be less successful in adapting to change, including hearing aid use.

Hearing aid studies have shown that people who have a positive outlook on life do better with hearing aids.[6] They have a positive self-image and believe they're in control of their life. My recommendation is take charge and be determined to improve the quality of your life with today's modern hearing aids!

4. Age of Your Hearing Aids

It is human nature to want to keep your hearing aids as long as possible in order to maximize value. However, it should be kept in mind that hearing aids do break down over time, ear canals change in shape, and your hearing loss is likely to change in time. In the research that I have conducted, customer satisfaction is at its highest in the first three months of use (69 percent). After five years of use, satisfaction drops significantly to 46 percent and after fifteen years of use even lower to 35 percent.[7]

So, it's important that you make sure that both the physical and audiological fit of your hearing aids is optimized for your hearing loss today rather than the way it was five, ten or fifteen years ago. I would recommend that you replace your hearing aids every four years; if your hearing aids are programmable you may be able to keep them longer since your hearing care provider can usually adjust them to the degree of hearing loss you currently have.

5. Choice of Technology

I have conducted extensive research across dozens of technologies. There is no doubt that customers are more satisfied with programmable technology.[3,8] Advanced programmable technology allows the dispenser to adjust the hearing aid to your specific hearing loss characteristics with more precision. If the product does not meet your needs then the hearing health professional can adjust the hearing aid at their location versus sending it back to the manufacturer for adjustment.

With advancements in hearing aid technology, there has been a corresponding improvement in computer software that acoustically fits your hearing instruments to your specific needs. For example, some manufacturers store hundreds of "real world" sounds in the computer and allow you to see how your hearing aids will sound in those situations. This tremendous feature allows the hearing aid dispenser to dynamically adjust the hearing aids based on your personal reaction to sounds. If you can afford advanced technology, do not hesitate to purchase programmable hearing aids.

A second advanced feature to consider is directional hearing aids. They have either two or three microphones in them. Because of their design they are able to reduce some annoying background noise and have been proven in both the lab and in the real world to improve your ability to understand speech in many difficult listening situations. I have conducted three studies on directional hearing aids. I found a 17 percent customer satisfaction improvement in two studies and a 26 percent improvement in another.[3,4,8] The latter achieved a 90 percent customer satisfaction rating, the highest I have ever seen in a hearing aid. If you are an active person, then directional hearing aids could be suitable for you.

6. Controls on Your Hearing Aid

Your goal is to purchase a hearing aid that never needs adjustments. It should graciously determine the volume you need and adjust its directionality by sensing if you are in quiet or a variety of noisy situations. If you have a completely digital hearing aid, when it comes across steady state noise like in an airplane cabin or around an air conditioner, it should improve your hearing comfort in these situations by making the sounds more tolerable. In addition, it should not give you feedback (whistling, buzzing or squealing) as it amplifies sounds around you. It should restore your ability to enjoy some soft sounds (e.g. leaves rustling, bubbling of a fish tank, etc.) while sensing very loud sounds and making them comfortable for you (loud sounds should never be painful to your ears).

While the industry has in principle developed automatic hearing instruments, some people need to personally control their hearing instruments. Research has shown, especially among experienced wearers, that some people (roughly a third) still need either a volume control, multiple memory switch (quiet versus noisy situation switch) or a remote control in order to control volume or to access different hearing aid strategies for handling different listening environments. Some people need control of their hearing aid for the following reasons: the automatic feature does not meet their needs in 100 percent of listening situations; psychologically the hearing aid wearer simply must have control of their hearing aids; or they are long-term hearing aid wearers who is used to a volume control and is therefore unwilling to part with it through habit.

It is very important that you determine your needs with respect to control of the hearing aid. You don't want to fiddle with your hearing aids every ten minutes but then again you don't want to be frustrated because your hearing aids work well in most situations but not in ten percent of your favorite situations (e.g. listening to soft music). This is an area that needs to be explored with your hearing health professional.

7. Sound Quality

One of the most important aspects of an enjoyable hearing aid experience is that you like the sound quality of hearing aids. So when you test-run your hearing aids, make sure that you consider the following dimensions of sound quality:

- Do you like the sound of your voice?
- Is the sound clean and crisp (sound clarity)?
- Is the sound too tinny?
- Does your hearing aid plug up your ears and muffle sound?
- Does it make some pleasant soft sounds audible to you?
- Are loud sounds uncomfortable to you?
- Are your hearing aids natural sounding?
- Does music sound pleasant and rich in texture?
- Does the world sound like you are in a barrel?
- Does your hearing aid whistle, buzz or squeal on its own?

With today's modern digital hearing aids, most of these problems should be solved. If you notice any of these problems during the trial run and in your follow-up visits, by all means talk to your hearing health professional about these issues. Such professionals are now capable of adjusting your hearing aids to your satisfaction. The extent to which all of the possible sound quality issues can be resolved is, of course, governed by the severity of your hearing loss. In other words, some types of hearing losses are simply more conducive to restoration of rich sound quality in many listening environments while others are not.

8. Do not Purchase Based Only on Cosmetics

Since the 1990s, the hearing aid industry has reduced the size of hearing aids to near invisibility. People can now wear them with greater comfort and we're finding very small CIC hearing aids have their distinct advantages such as on the telephone and in outdoor situations. Some people are concerned with cosmetics and prefer the least noticeable hearing aids, in the way that you might choose contact lenses instead of framed eyeglasses. The problem is that the smallest hearing aid may not be the most suitable hearing solution for you for a variety of reasons. Your specific hearing loss may require more power than is available in CICs.

Because of hearing loss stigma or embarrassment, many

consumers come into hearing healthcare offices and start off the dialog with, "I would like one of those invisible hearing aids that I saw on TV." A likely response may be something like: "We carry invisible hearing aids, but I first need to examine your ears, measure your hearing loss, assess your lifestyle and manual dexterity and then discuss how your hearing loss is impacting the quality of your life. You may or may not be a candidate for these hearing aids." If it is determined that you are not a candidate for CIC hearing aids and you still insist on buying them, the professional hearing health provider will not fit you with the product because in essence they would be giving you the wrong prescription for your hearing loss.

9. Have Realistic Expectations During the Trial Period

Follow the instructions you are given during the initial stages of adjustment. These are designed to help in formulating realistic expectations of what to expect from your hearing aids. You may need a specific wearing schedule for hearing aids. One experienced in-the-canal hearing aid wearer obtained CIC instruments a few years ago. He was in his early 30s and had used hearing aids since he was a teenager. When he returned for his two-week recheck, he was asked how long he could wear the instruments in the beginning. He said that he could only use them for fifteen minutes at a time. Within two weeks he was wearing them full-time and they were completely comfortable. Had he not been counseled that the deep insertion of the shell tip with CIC hearing aids may take extra time to fully adjust to, he might have become discouraged and given up on that particular style of hearing aids.

Be patient with yourself. If you have the best hearing aids for your hearing loss and your lifestyle, hang in there. Make sure you're comfortable with the advice you've been given. Ask questions. Remember, your provider is your advocate. Satisfied hearing aid wearers are not shy when it comes to telling others about their success, but unfortunately, neither are the ones who are dissatisfied. No two people are alike, and it's not a good idea to assume if someone has had a bad experience, all hearing aids are bad. You could very well be one of the overwhelming majority who has a good experience! There are many reasons why someone may not have been successful, so don't project these conditions and improbabilities onto yourself. Also, do not expect someone else's hearing aids to work for you. Would you wear their eyeglasses and decide whether you could be helped based on this experience?

Be realistic. Hearing aids will not permit you to hear the flapping of hummingbird wings over a lawnmower. Remember that it takes time to get used to hearing aids, especially if you're a new wearer. Keep in mind that background noise is almost always part of your environment, and adjustment to it is required. In time, you will tune out many of these everyday sounds. It's important not to become disappointed or frustrated while your brain begins to adjust to a whole new world of sound. If you're an experienced wearer trying new hearing aids, understand that they might not sound like your old ones. Before you reject them, allow neural hook-ups in the auditory system to adapt to these new sounds. You just might find that you like this new sound better than the old one.

10. Earwax Protection

One of the common causes of hearing aid failure is that moisture and earwax fill up the receiver tubing of the hearing aid causing the hearing aid speaker to no longer function correctly.

I strongly suggest that you purchase hearing aids with proven methods of keeping earwax out of the hearing aid. I have personally studied more than 90,000 hearing aid owners over a two-year period and determined that it is possible to reduce hearing aid repairs by 50 percent due to receiver failure by using a wax guard at the end of the hearing aids.[9]

12 Reasons to Purchase Two Hearing Aids Instead of One

Research with more than 5,000 consumers with hearing loss in both ears demonstrated that binaurally fit subjects (two hearing aids) are more satisfied than those monaurally fit (one hearing aid).[10]

When given the choice and allowed to hear binaurally, the overwhelming majority of consumers choose two hearing aids over one.

Consequently, binaural users tend to communicate better in their place of worship, in small group gatherings, large gatherings and even outdoors. Naturally, a person's ability to enjoy hearing aids will differ based on the specific hearing loss and the type of technology used in the hearing aids.

Nevertheless, if you have a hearing loss in both ears and there is useable hearing in your poorer ear, budget permitting, I would recommend a hearing aid for both ears. Many hearing healthcare providers can demonstrate the binaural advantage on your very first visit, under headphone testing or even with a programmable fitting.

Based on a review of the literature and my own research with thousands of consumers with hearing loss in both ears, here are many reasons why you should purchase a binaural hearing system when two are indicated.[11]

1. Keeps both ears active, resulting in less hearing deterioration. As Dr. Carmen identifies in Chapter One, research has shown that when only one hearing instrument is worn, the unaided ear tends to lose its ability to hear and understand. This is clinically called the auditory deprivation effect. People wearing two hearing instruments keep both ears active. In fact, wearing one hearing aid (when two are indicated) could result in greater deterioration of hearing in the unaided ear than if wearing no hearing aid at all.

2. Better understanding of speech. By wearing two hearing instruments rather than one, selective listening is more easily achieved. This means your brain can focus on the conversation you want to hear. Research shows that people wearing two hearing aids routinely understand speech and conversation significantly better than people wearing one.

3. Better understanding in group and noisy situations. Speech intelligibility is improved in difficult listening situations when wearing two hearing aids. However, advanced binaural technology (programmable analog or digital) tends to perform better in noise than older (analog) technology.

4. Better ability to tell direction of sound. This is called localization. Research shows that in binaural use, there's an average of a 15 percent shift in increased satisfaction in "ability to tell the direction of sounds." This is a substantial improvement! In a social gathering, for example, localization allows you to hear from which direction someone is speaking to you. In traffic, you can tell from which direction a car or siren is coming.

5. Better sound quality. When you listen to a stereo system, you use both speakers to get the smoothest, sharpest, most natural sound quality. The same thing can be said of hearing aids. By wearing two hearing instruments, you increase your hearing range from 180 degrees reception (with just one instrument) to 360 degrees. This greater range provides a better sense of balance and sound quality.

6. Smoother tone quality. Wearing two hearing instruments generally requires less volume. This results in less distortion and better reproduction of sounds.

7. Reduced feedback and whistling. With a lower volume control setting the chances of hearing aid feedback is reduced.

8. Wider hearing range. It's true. A person can hear sounds from a further distance with two ears, rather than just one. A voice that's barely heard at ten feet with one ear can be heard up to forty feet with two ears.

9. Better sound identification. Often, with just one hearing instrument, many noises and words sound alike. But with two hearing instruments, as with two ears, sounds are more easily distinguishable.

10. Hearing is less tiring and listening more pleasant. More binaural hearing aid wearers report that listening and participating in conversation is more enjoyable with two instruments. This is because you do not have to strain to hear with the better ear. Thus, binaural hearing can help make listening (and therefore life) more relaxing.

11. Feeling of balanced hearing. Two-eared hearing results in a feeling of balanced reception of sound, also known as the stereo effect, whereas monaural hearing creates an unusual feeling of sounds being heard in one ear.

12. Tinnitus Masking. About 50 percent of people with ringing in their ears report improvement when wearing hearing aids. If you have a hearing aid in only one ear, there will still be ringing in the unaided ear.

How to Align Your Expectations
with Hearing Aid Performance

Here are some issues you should keep in mind as you develop appropriate expectations about what your hearing aids can and cannot do for you:[12-13]

- No matter how technically advanced, in most cases hearing aids cannot restore your hearing to normal except is some very mild hearing losses.
- Not all hearing aids perform the same with every type of hearing loss.
- No hearing aid has been designed which will filter out all background noise. Some hearing instruments can reduce amplification of some types of background noise or make you more comfortable in the presence of noise.
- Where appropriate, directional microphones can often improve your ability to hear in noise.
- When directional hearing instruments are coupled with digital signal processing, you can be assured that your hearing instruments are optimized for improving your quality of life in noisy environments.
- Since you are purchasing custom hearing instruments, you should expect the fit to be comfortable; ideally you should not even know they are in your ears. There should not be any soreness, bleeding, or rashes associated with your wearing hearing aids. If there is, go back to your hearing health provider to make adjustments to the shell of the aid or earmold.
- Hearing instruments should allow you to:
  (1) hear soft sounds (e.g. child's voice, soft speech) that you could not hear without amplification—this is part of the enjoyment of hearing aids;
  (2) understand speech in quiet situations—many people will derive some additional speech intelligibility in noise with advanced technology;
  (3) prevent loud sounds from becoming uncomfortably loud for you, but very loud sounds that are uncomfortable to normal hearing people may still be uncomfortable to you.
- Hearing aids may squeal or whistle when you are inserting them into your ear (if you do not have a volume control to

shut it off); but if it squeals after the initial insertion, then most likely you have an inadequate fit and should tell your hearing health provider.

- Do not expect your friend's hearing aid brand or style to work for you.

- Do not expect your family doctor to know very much about hearing loss, brands of hearing aids and whether or not you need them.

- Expect your hearing aids to provide benefit to you during the trial period. By benefit, I mean that your ability to understand speech has demonstrably improved in the listening situations important to you (with realistic expectations though). This is what you paid for, so you should expect benefit. If you do not experience an improvement, then work with your hearing health professional to see if the instrument can be adjusted to meet your specific needs. Never purchase a hearing aid that does not give you sufficient benefit.

- Expect to be satisfied with your hearing instruments; expect the quality of your life to improve due to your hearing instruments.

- Expect a 30-day trial period with a money-back guarantee if your hearing aids do not give you benefit. (There might be a small nonrefundable portion for some services rendered.)

- Give your hearing aids a chance, being sure to follow the instructions of the hearing health provider. Most people need a period of adjustment (called acclimatization) before they are deriving the maximum benefit from their hearing instruments (even up to four months).

Common Myths about Hearing Loss and Hearing Aids

There are many common myths still prevalent about hearing loss and hearing aids. I would like to dispel these myths now that you are living in the 21st Century.

Your hearing loss cannot be helped.

In the past, many people with hearing loss in one ear, with a high frequency hearing loss, or with nerve damage have all been told they cannot be helped, often by their family practice physician. This might have been true many years ago, but with modern advances in technology, nearly 95 percent of people with a sensorineural hearing loss *can* be helped with hearing aids.

Hearing loss affects only "old people" and is merely a sign of aging.

Only 35 percent of people with hearing loss are older than age 64. There are close to six million people in the U.S. between the ages of 18 and 44 with hearing loss, and more than one million are school age. Hearing loss affects all age groups.

If I had a hearing loss, my family doctor would have told me.

Not true! Only 14 percent of physicians routinely screen for hearing loss during a physical. Since most hearing-impaired people hear well in a quiet environment like your doctor's office, it can be virtually impossible for your physician to recognize the extent of your problem. Without special training in, and understanding of the nature of hearing loss, it may be difficult for your doctor to even believe that you have a hearing problem.

The consequences of hiding hearing loss are better than wearing hearing aids.

What price are you paying for vanity? I go back to the old adage that an untreated hearing loss is far more noticeable than hearing aids. If you miss a punch line to a joke, or respond inappropriately in conversation, people may have concerns about your mental acuity, your attention span or your ability to communicate effectively. The personal consequences of vanity can be life altering. At a simplistic level, untreated hearing loss means giving up some of the pleasant sounds you used to enjoy. At a deeper level, vanity could severely reduce the quality of your life.

Only people with serious hearing loss need hearing aids.

The need for hearing amplification is dependent on your lifestyle, your need for refined hearing, and the degree of your hearing loss. If you are a lawyer, teacher or a group psychotherapist, where very refined hearing is necessary to discern the nuances of human communication, then even a mild hearing loss can be intolerable. If you live in a rural area by yourself and seldom socialize, then perhaps you are someone who is tolerant of even moderate hearing losses.

I'll just have some minor surgery like my friend did, and then my hearing will be okay.

Many people know someone whose hearing improved after medical or surgical treatment, and it's true that some types of hearing loss can be successfully treated. With adults, unfortunately, this only applies to five to ten percent of cases.

My hearing loss is normal for my age.

Isn't this a strange way to look at things? But, do you realize that well-meaning doctors tell this to their patients everyday. It happens to be "normal" for overweight people to have high blood pressure. That doesn't mean they should not receive treatment for the problem.

I have one ear that's down a little, but the other one's okay.

Everything is relative. Nearly all patients who believe that they have one "good" ear actually have two "bad" ears. When one ear is slightly better than the other, we learn to favor that ear for the telephone, group conversations, and so forth. It can give the illusion that "the better ear" is normal when it isn't. Most types of hearing loss affect both ears fairly equally, and about 90 percent of patients are in need of hearing aids for both ears.

Hearing aids will make me look "older" and "handicapped."

Looking older is clearly more affected by almost all other factors besides hearing aids. It's not the hearing aids that make one look older, it's what one may believe they imply. If hearing aids help you function like a normal hearing person, for all intents and purposes, the stigma is removed. Hearing aid manufacturers are well aware that cosmetics are an issue to many people, and that's why today we have hearing aids that fit totally in the ear canal (essentially not noticeable unless someone is staring directly into your ear). This CIC style of hearing aid has enough power and special features to satisfy at least 50 percent of individuals with hearing impairment. But more importantly, keep in mind that "a hearing loss is more obvious than a hearing aid." Smiling and nodding your head when you don't understand what's being said makes your condition more apparent than the largest hearing aid.

Hearing aids will make everything sound too loud.

Hearing aids are amplifiers. At one time, the way that hearing aids were designed, it was necessary to turn up the power in order to hear soft speech (or other soft sounds). Then, normal conversation indeed would have been too loud. With today's hearing aids, however, the circuit works automatically, only providing the amount of amplification needed based on the input level. In fact, many hearing aids today don't have a volume control.

Conclusions

Hopefully, you now recognize the value of hearing aids and the significant impact they can have on your life, as well as the life of your family and associates. I also hope you realize that hearing aids may not necessarily be an instant cure for your hearing difficulties, but with patience, you will find they can be your bridge to healing.

Enjoy the experience!

References

1. Kochkin S. MarkeTrak V: Why my hearing aids are in the drawer: the consumer's perspective. The Hearing Journal 53(2): 34-42, 2000.
2. Kochkin S. MarkeTrak IV: correlates of hearing aid purchase intent. The Hearing Journal 51(1): 30-41, 1998.
3. Kochkin S. Customer satisfaction and subjective benefit with high-performance hearing instruments. The Hearing Review 3(12): 16-26, 1996.
4. Kochkin S. MarkeTrak VI – 10 year customer satisfaction trends in the U.S. hearing instrument market. The Hearing Review 9(10): 14-25, 46, 2003.
5. Kochkin S and Rogin C. Quantifying the obvious: the impact of hearing aids on quality of life, The Hearing Review 6(1): 8-34, 2000.
6. Singer J, Healey J. and Preece J. Hearing instruments: a psychological and behavioral perspective. High Performance Hearing Solutions 1, 1997.
7. Kochkin S. MarkeTrak VI database, Knowles Electronics: Itasca, IL. (Unpublished).
8. Kochkin S. Customer satisfaction with single and multiple microphone digital hearing aids, The Hearing Review 7(11): 24-29, 2000.

9. Kochkin S. Finally a solution to the cerumen problem. The Hearing Review: 9(4): 2002.

10. Kochkin S. and Kuk F. The binaural advantage: evidence from subjective benefit and customer satisfaction data. The Hearing Review:4(4): 29,30-32,34, 1997.

11. Kochkin S. *Binaural Hearing Aids: The Fitting of Choice for Bilateral Loss Subjects.* (An unpublished technical paper.) Itasca, IL: Knowles Electronics, 2000.

12. Allen, Rose. Reasonable Expectations for the Consumer. www.healthyhearing.com. August, 2002.

13. Stypulkowski P. Realistic expectations: a key to success. High Performance Hearing Solutions 1, 1997.

CHAPTER EIGHT
The Questions and Answers
What the Experts Say
Richard Carmen, Au.D.

Dr. Carmen received his Doctor of Audiology Degree from the Arizona School of Health Sciences, a division of the Kirksville College of Osteopathic Medicine. He's been practicing audiology and issuing hearing aids since 1972, during which time he pioneered research into the effects of metabolic diseases on hearing. He has written extensively in the field as a regular contributor to various hearing journals, and of his previous book publications, two were written for the consumer. His material has appeared in such popular consumer-based periodicals as *The Saturday Evening Post, Ladies' Home Journal* and *Self Magazine*. He has maintained his present clinical practice in Sedona, Arizona since 1990.

While this book strives to address the most important issues pertaining to hearing loss and hearing aids, this section covers questions and answers not addressed elsewhere in this book. The questions developed were ones you yourself may have wanted to ask. As a result, the most seasoned and tenured professionals were invited to answer them. Here's what the experts had to say!

1. From your research, what have you discovered about the process of *listening*?

Richard Halley, Ph.D., Professor of Communication at Weber State University, Ogden, Utah, is considered an expert on the topic of listening. He has been a longtime board member of the International Listening Association and has written many papers and a few books on this subject matter. Among newsworthy attention directed to Dr. Halley's work, he has been a repeated guest on ABC's "20/20."

The most obvious connection between hearing and listening is that if one does not hear the sounds, we cannot expect that person to interpret the meaning of the sounds with any accuracy. One of the things we know about listening is that people tend to hear what they want to hear (or more accurately what they expect to hear). Each individual literally creates in their mind a fairly accurate mathematical model of what they expect a message to be like. This capacity makes it possible for us to predict something about what a person is likely to say.

130

The advantage is that often when we're listening and we don't hear a small part of a sentence, we can guess quite accurately at what the rest of the sentence is. However, if you lose some hearing, you still have the mathematical models in your head and the predictions for what comes next in a message remain pretty strong. Yet, if you're not hearing accurately or are missing some of the sounds (some of the words even), your capacity to accurately predict is greatly reduced. If you have a hearing loss, you must learn to be conscious of the effects it has on your ability to predict. If you're careful, prediction can help you understand because your brain often knows how to fill in some of the missing parts. But if you assume this process is still as accurate as it was before your hearing loss, and you interpret messages based on what was heard with the old models, the number of interpretation errors you make will increase dramatically.

One of the things we know is that men and women process information differently. Thus, it's important that we not talk as though all of our advice will work exactly the same for both sexes. One of the major differences is that men better than women are often able to stay focused on one speaker and ignore others in the environment. This has the advantage that many men may be able to work in situations that are noisier than many women can tolerate. It has the significant disadvantage that men often do not hear someone call to them when they are concentrating on a message such as a TV program, or more specifically, like Monday night football! This is true for men with good hearing. If you are hard of hearing, listening becomes that much more difficult.

On the other hand, women far more often than men tend to check their environment for other important messages. The advantage is that women can often work on one task and be able to check another task often enough that they can also complete the second task. For example, many women can fix dinner or work on some other task while staying aware of a small child without putting the youngster at risk. Their multi-focus ability exceeds that of men. The disadvantage is that when women listen to a message that requires a great deal of concentration (perhaps because the material is new or difficult), they will still check their environment for other messages and may miss critical parts of that difficult message and thus become confused or misunderstand the message.

So, listening requires focus despite your gender, and whether you have good hearing or not. Hearing loss merely makes the listening process more challenging.

2. Is there a relationship between *exercise* and *better hearing*?

Helaine Alessio, Ph.D. Professor, Department of Physical Health, Health and Sports Studies at Miami University, is a Fellow of the American College of Sports Medicine and a Scripps Gerontology Fellow, and the recipient of several NIH grants.

Kathleen Hutchinson, Ph.D., Professor and Chair, Department of Speech Pathology and Audiology at Miami University, is Chair of the Department of Speech Pathology and Audiology, and has authored several articles on personality attributes related to hearing aid use and aural rehabilitation.

Dr. Alessio and Dr. Hutchinson have co-authored more than twenty research papers and are currently working on a longitudinal study on cardiovascular health and hearing sensitivity.

In plain English, Yes! Recent advances in medicine and positive changes toward healthy lifestyles have challenged some long held assumptions about "inevitable aging changes"—including hearing loss. Impaired hearing in older years has always been considered as something to be expected. Although significant hearing loss is present in approximately 1 out of every 3 Americans aged 65 years and older, we've learned that hearing sensitivity can be maintained very well into those "older" years if:

- you were not exposed to loud noises at work or home for long periods of time;
- you wore ear protection when exposed to loud noises;
- you did not take certain ototoxic medications;
- and if you maintained a healthy cardiovascular fitness level.

The exception to these findings would be a hearing loss with a genetic component or a family history of hearing impairment. Research from our laboratory and several others in the U.S. have consistently reported a positive relation between the cardiovascular system and functional ability of the organs and tissues in the inner ear. Much of the explanation behind the protective effects of cardiovascular fitness lies in enhanced circulation of blood that is needed to supply the bones and muscles of the inner ear. When blood flow is impeded, then nutrients (like antioxidants and protective heat shock proteins) will not be available. Blood flow can be impeded by cholesterol build-up in the walls of the artery, and vasoconstriction (narrowing) that has been correlated with high blood pressure, smoking, stress, and some personality types.

The U.S. Surgeon General's report on *Physical Activity and Health* recommends that everyone engage in aerobic exercise. Figure 8-1 shows the benefits to aerobic exercise in most age groups when cardiovascular fitness is attained.

132

This means large muscle movements, such as walking, bicycling, and swimming, for at least 20-30 minutes at a time, five days per week. When examining exercise that is performed on a one-time only basis, aerobic exercise may divert blood flow from metabolically less active parts of the body (like organs and tissues of the inner ear) to metabolically more active parts (like skeletal muscles engaged in exercise). This may at first appear to be harmful. However, exercise on a regular basis has been shown to result in blood that is well-stocked with nutrients (like vitamins, antioxidants, and adequate levels of sugar), protective proteins (like heat shock proteins), as well as blood that is not littered with cholesterol, triglycerides, or too much sugar.

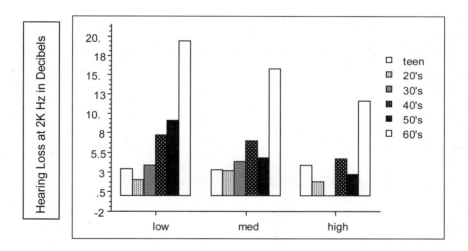

Figure 8-1: The higher the cardiovascular fitness, the better hearing in most age groups.

When performed regularly, aerobic exercise results in blood vessels that tend to be more supple, allowing for transitions in blood flow from rest to exercise, and resilient to withstanding blood pressure changes without suffering major impairments to the walls of the arteries. These changes to the vessels that carry blood impact every square inch of the body because cells live or die by blood supply and debris removal.

Our research during the past decade on over a thousand subjects ages 8-88 have resulted in the following conclusions:

1) hearing loss occurs with age, but noticeable hearing loss does not appear until after age 50;

2) having low cardiovascular fitness at any age is associated with poorer hearing sensitivity compared to those with medium or high level cardiovascular fitness; and

3) persons older than 50 who have moderate or high cardiovascular fitness levels maintain their hearing sensitivity comparable to persons who are in their 30's.

We speculate that the association of hearing loss and cardiovascular fitness are related by the common mechanism of improved blood circulation.

3. We know that the heart carries nutrition throughout the body, including the ear. Without absorption of nutrients critical to hearing, its function would stop. For example, many people who have gone on a starvation diet as a political protest have lost some of their hearing. Since Americans have become so vitamin and mineral conscious, is there anything you can recommend that has been shown to positively impact hearing?

Martin Dayton, D.O., is Past-President of the International and American Association of Clinical Nutritionists. Dr. Dayton is in clinical practice in Miami, Florida.

Unfortunately, no specific nutritional treatment is generally used or known to address hearing loss in all people. However, strategies do exist which may address the needs of the individual with impaired hearing, in accordance with the unique circumstances of the person. These circumstances are governed by the inherited and acquired strengths and weaknesses of the individual and the conditions under which the person exists.

A child may have an inherited predisposition to allergies and live in an environment where junk food is a staple. This child may be prone to develop a form of "stuffed ears" known as serous otitis media. Fluid accumulates in the middle ear due to allergy-mediated inflammation, swelling, and closure of the Eustachian tube. Dysfunctional pressures may develop in the ear. Infection may take hold in part due to impaired transport of immune factors to the area and impaired drainage of toxic fluids from the ear due to swelling.

On the other hand, an elderly person with an inherited predisposition to hardening of the arteries who eats the nutritionally sub-optimal standard American diet may develop progressive hearing loss. This is due to auditory nerve tissue deterioration associated with impaired circulation—accelerated with aging. Perhaps, accumulation of environmental or pharmaceutical toxic materials with time is also a role in the manifestation of hearing loss.

These two cases illustrate how diverse the contributing circumstances can be in regard to the manifestation of hearing loss. Each case must be handled differently in the use of nutrition to address the same goal of improved hearing. The child in the first example needs to avoid foods which may trigger allergies. Wheat, cow's milk, peanuts, chocolate, eggs, and soy are frequent offenders. Various methods are used to determine which foods need to be avoided, when and how often. Various methods may be used to reduce such sensitivities. Plant extracts from stinging nettles, aloe vera, citrus and seeds of grapes may reverse the allergic processes. Vitamins, such as C and pantothenic acid may also be useful. Addressing deficiencies of various substances improves overall resistance to disease.

The older person in the second example needs to improve circulation and, in part, to reverse processes which lead to deterioration. Plant extracts such as Ginkgo biloba improves efficiency and function of tissues subject to sub-optimal circulation. Niacin increases blood flow via dilation of blood vessels and may restore cholesterol to a more optimal state. Turmeric (Curcuma longa) reduces the tendency to build-up of blockages within the walls of arteries, and helps prevent deterioration of tissues.

Various substances help prevent tissue deterioration and foster repair. Optimal repair of nerve tissue needs an abundance of the components found in such tissue cofactors which make them work. Lecithin contains materials needed for cell wall repair, and chemicals needed for communication between nerve cells. Vitamin B12, alpha-lipoic acid, and thiamin are co-factors that help maintain and repair nerve tissue. Various nutritional substances help to directly remove toxins, or fortify the detoxification organs of the body so they are more effective in achieving their intended purpose. Adequate detoxification is necessary for normal function and repair. Vitamin C, garlic, and chlorella, are helpful. And many nutritional substances have multiple benefits.

Animal and plant substances may be used in various ways. For example, extracts from fetal (unborn young) sheep tissues, such as from the fetal auditory nerve, may be taken by injection to stimulate organization and regeneration of human tissues associated with hearing. Fetal tissue is programmed by nature to generate into fully functioning organ systems. After peak reproductive years, bodily tissues are programmed to disorganize and deteriorate to eventually make room for the next generations to come. The use of fetal tissue appears, in part, to counter this trend.

The most important aspect of nutritional care in regard to ear problems lies between the ears in taking care of the needs of the rest of the person who is attached to the ears.

4. Most of us would assume, once hair cells die, the condition is permanent with irreversible sensorineural hearing loss. Would you share with readers what you've discovered, and any implications it might hold for restoration of hearing in humans?

Edwin W Rubel, Ph.D., is Virginia Merrill Bloedel Professor of Hearing Science, and Professor in the Departments of Otolaryngology—Head and Neck Surgery, Physiology/Biophysics, Neurological Surgery and Psychology at the University of Washington. Dr. Rubel has published over 200 scientific articles and edited three books on various topics related to development and plasticity of the auditory system.

Research on hair cell regeneration was not a major topic of research in hearing science until 1986-87. At that time, my group was one of two that discovered mature birds had the remarkable natural ability to reform their inner ear hair cells. This occurred after either damage produced by loud noises or after damage produced by certain therapeutic drugs like antibiotics (see Figure 8-2). This was quite startling to us as well as to the rest of the scientific community. Confirmation through DNA technology supported what we were seeing. After damage occurred, there were indeed new hair cells generated by renewed cell division in several species of fully mature birds.

We now know that all vertebrates, *except mammals*, can regenerate new hair cells in the inner ear after native hair cells are damaged or destroyed. In some parts of the inner ear of some animals, there is ongoing production and death of hair cells (like the "turnover" of skin cells) throughout life, while in others new cells are produced only when there is damage to the native ones. We and others are working hard to understand the molecular chain of events responsible for hair cell regeneration in the species where it occurs. This may provide the clues for how to make it happen in humans and other mammals.

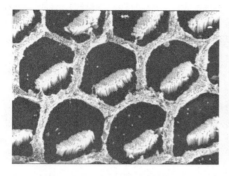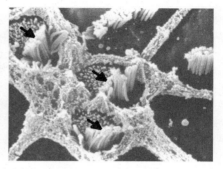

Photomicrographs provided courtesy of Edwin W. Rubel, Ph.D., Virginia Merrill Bloedel Hearing Research Center, University of Washington. Used by permission.

Figure 8-2: Left photo shows normal hair cell clusters. Right photo arrows show hair cell regeneration after being destroyed.

The work on mammals now is at a point where we can induce a small amount of cell division in the inner ear in a dish (that is, in culture), as well as in vivo (occurring within a living organism). This has been done on mice, guinea pigs and rats using a variety of growth-promoting molecules. We have also discovered one gene (and there will be others) that is responsible for turning off the production of hair cells during development and may be involved in preventing regeneration.

Therefore, we at least know that it's *possible* to induce the first stage of regeneration to a limited extent in the inner ear sensory epithelium of mature mammals. The sensory epithelia make up parts of the inner ear that cause the initial response to sound and balance. So, most of the success has been done in the balance parts of the inner ear, but we and others are working on the cochlea. In fact, a team of researchers has recently used new findings from research on development of the inner ear to induce a few new cells in the guinea pig cochlea to become hair cells, again proving that it will be possible.

The good news is that for the first time in history, there are teams of investigators worldwide exploring the possibility that hair cell regeneration can be induced in the mammal and human cochlea. In the mid-1990s, there were only two laboratories exploring this possibility. Now there are probably 20 or 30. The bad news is funding. It's a real problem. Until we actually find candidate molecules for use in humans, this research won't be taken over by pharmaceutical companies. Once they step in, they will heavily invest in developing human therapies. But, until then, the entire cost of this research must be borne by the federal government and private foundations.

I feel that within five to ten years, we could easily find out if it's possible to regenerate hair cells at robust levels, sufficient to restore hearing in mammals if the funds were available to support large multi-investigator teams working on this problem. Unfortunately, such funding does not exist at this time so small groups are struggling along to get one grant after another and do one experiment at a time. From discovery of molecules that could induce regeneration in laboratory animals, it could be as little as another 10 years until we achieve hair cell regeneration in humans. If successful, it could eliminate some of the need for hearing aids and cochlear implants as we now know them.

When I started this work, somebody said to me that I'd never be able to restore the complexity and intricacies of hair cells in humans or other mammals. My response hasn't changed: "You could be right, but without trying, it surely won't happen. If our goal is to actually restore hearing—it's the only game in town."

5. How can we change present prejudices and misunderstanding about hearing loss and the use of hearing aids?

Ray P. Cuzzort, Ph.D., Boulder, Colorado. Dr. Cuzzort has taught sociology at the University of Colorado in Boulder for the past 30 years. As a leading Sociologist, he's written extensively on social theory, and published books and articles on this subject matter, specifically focusing on how people deal with stigmatic conditions.

I can answer this best by asking another set of questions: hearing aids have been shunned by a number of people with serious hearing problems, while eyeglasses are often worn by people with no meaningful loss of vision. Why is a prosthetic device avoided in one instance and welcomed in the other?

The foremost concern with any prosthetic device is how effectively it deals with the physical defect it seeks to correct. This is a relative matter and not as simple as it might first appear to be. If a defect is seriously debilitating, a moderately effective prosthetic device will be relied on. However, if a defect is modest, only a superbly effective prosthetic device is likely to be preferred by a wearer. Complicating the issue is the extent to which revealing the defect is considered stigmatizing by the person involved. If the defect is not seriously stigmatizing, then a prosthetic device is more likely to be utilized. For example, teenagers wear dental braces despite their mildly disfiguring appearance because ill-formed teeth are not seriously stigmatizing. Wearing a hearing aid, however, suggests that the wearer could be socially handicapped.

People commonly wear glasses when they don't need them. Sunglasses are worn in dark cafes by men and women who want to look "hip." Similarly, "bop" glasses are worn by ghetto youngsters who want to look like jazz musicians. The obvious point being made here is that glasses are not only a prosthetic device, but a stylistic one—a part of one's attire, so to speak. Like any other item of attire, glasses can enhance the image one is trying to project. They can also detract from it.

Another consideration to deal with is the folk history of a prosthetic device and how that history is perceived by the person faced with using the device. What associations does such a history bring to mind? For one thing, glasses are associated with intellectuals, office clerks, and bookish people. These are not strong positive associations, nor are they terribly negative ones either. Glasses don't threaten the image an individual is trying to sustain.

In light of the above comments, we can turn our attention to hearing aids. Its history, for many people, goes back to a time when a huge, trumpet-like device was waved by a crotchety old person in the direction of someone talking. It was commonly used by women in the advanced stages of senility. Note: this perception does not have to be accurate—it only has to exist in order to have some effect. (For both functional reasons and to rid the hearing aid of this onus, its design has moved quickly toward extremely small and relatively-easy-to-hide versions.)

Glasses have no age-specific associations, but hearing aids are seen as an indication of the infirmities that come with being older. In modern America, protests to the contrary, being old is a problem with respect to being stigmatized. It's very likely the case that when an individual is confronted with the choice of being stigmatized by a prosthetic device or being helped by it, avoidance of the stigma will be equally, or more important, as the value of the device. At the same time, it should also be recognized that stigmatization is a social creation. What is stigmatizing in one social context is not necessarily stigmatizing in another. (The classic example of this is the jagged facial scar that means one thing if it comes from an automobile accident and another if it comes from a duel of honor.) If this is so, then shifting attitudes toward aging as a stigmatizing condition will possibly bring about shifting attitudes toward the use of amplification.

Any campaigns toward changing public perception of hearing aids might consider the following possibilities. First, show more young people, even children, in situations where hearing aids are of benefit. More broadly, show people of varied ages and in different social contexts who are relying on hearing aids.

Second, provide specific and compelling measures of the effectiveness of hearing aids. This is a primary concern in any campaign to improve acceptance.

Third, direct some attention to the non-hearing aid wearer. Social interactions, even of a very informal nature, are stressful. If hearing aid wearers are convinced that people will shun them because they have hearing problems, they will be more likely either to put their hearing aids aside, or avoid people. If hearing aid wearers can be persuaded that non-hearing aid users are not inclined to perceive them as stigmatized, then the hearing aid will be more acceptable.

Fourth, in a modern social context in which a variety of physical handicaps have been granted more tolerant social perceptions, deafness should be defined as a condition that can be effectively dealt with by the use of hearing aids, by sensitivity on the part of all involved with those who are hearing-impaired, and by a willingness on the part of the hearing-impaired person to remain a participating member of the human community.

6. Most people have heard of the condition of Meniere's Disease, but few, including those suffering from it, have a good understanding of the problem. Can you help clarify this disorder, and how it might differ from the similar condition of labyrinthitis?

Dennis Poe, M.D., Massachusetts Eye and Ear, Boston. Dr. Poe is an otolaryngologist specializing in neurotologic surgery and is Editor of, and Contributor to *The Consumer Handbook on Dizziness and Vertigo* (Auricle Ink Publishers, 2005). He is a Past-Board member of the Prosper Meniere's Society and considered a foremost expert on Meniere's Disease.

Dizziness and balance disorders are very common and rank among the most frequent problems seen on a daily basis by health care providers of all types. The most common causes of sudden vertigo or imbalance are Vestibular Neuritis, an inflammation or irritation of the balance nerve, Labyrinthitis, inflammation or irritation of the inner ear, Migraines, causing reduced blood flow to the balance centers in the brain, and Meniere's Disease, a disruption of the inner ear due to fluid swelling. Labyrinthitis and Meniere's Disease may be associated with varying degrees of hearing loss.

Medical professionals define vertigo as any hallucination of movement when in fact no real movement has occurred. The most common form of this is the spinning sensation that results after rapidly rotating oneself and stopping quickly. If vertigo is severe enough, it can cause secondary symptoms of nausea, vomiting, and cold sweats. It's estimated that about one third of the population will experience a significant bout of sudden vertigo during their lifetime, and the vast majority of these are due to vestibular neuritis or labyrinthitis. Still, Meniere's is common enough to affect as many as one out of 50 individuals.

Vestibular neuritis is presumably caused by viral inflammation of the vestibular (balance) nerve that brings inner ear information to the brain and results in vertigo and balance disturbances without hearing loss. More severe cases may also damage hearing or the cochlear nerve. Viral inflammation of the inner ear itself is called Labyrinthitis and usually causes both vertigo and hearing loss. Severe cases of neuritis or labyrinthitis can cause sudden unexpected vertiginous attacks with a complete loss of balance that is made worse by any head movements or by watching anything move.

These symptoms can often last for hours causing nausea, vomiting, sometimes diarrhea, all of which can be a profoundly frightening experience. The episodes are usually quite harmless and completely resolve on their own in a few days without any treatment. Like many viral illnesses, it normally will not recur. More severe forms may cause a few after shock spells of lesser magnitude within a few days of the original attack. Once the acute vertigo attacks have subsided, there's a period of dysequilibrium—a sensation that the balance is off, and may last for hours, days, or many weeks, depending on the severity of the attacks. Treatment is usually limited to symptom relief with medications to quiet the balance system. A regular exercise program is recommended to speed up the recovery process after the balance injury by stimulating the natural process of *vestibular compensation.*

Even if some degree of permanent injury were to have occurred, the brain can use information from the injured balance organ or nerve and combine it with information from the normal side. The new balance signals are integrated with the vision and senses of position and feeling in the limbs to recreate an effective balance system. Exercising speeds up this compensation process.

Meniere's Disease is believed to be the long-term result of an injury to the labyrinth, such as severe labyrinthitis that has failed to heal properly and has gone on to become a recurring cause of vertigo attacks and hearing injury. Symptoms of Meniere's Disease include recurring vertigo attacks, fluctuating hearing loss, abnormal noises in the ear (tinnitus), and pressure or fullness in the ear. This can be caused by a condition known as endolymphatic hydrops (swelling of the endolymph). This is the fluid that fills the innermost compartment of the inner ear. The excessive pressure is believed to result from a breakdown in the pressure-regulating mechanisms and can be simplistically likened to water on the knee years after an injury. When the inner ear fluids swell, it causes some strain that initially may be mistaken for pressure in the middle ear, as might be experienced with infections, or airplane travel. If the swelling continues, hearing loss, especially in the lower frequencies, may fluctuate and be associated with tinnitus, the warning noises the ear creates when injured.

Ultimately, unprovoked episodes of spinning vertigo can develop, sometimes even waking someone from sleep with a violent sense of rotation, nausea, and vomiting. The attack can last for minutes or hours and usually subsides, leaving the person exhausted and very unstable with significant dysequilibrium for many more hours, days, or even weeks, going through the same vestibular compensation recovery as occurs after a labyrinthitis spell.

Meniere's is much more disabling because these spells recur unexpectedly and with variable frequency, creating a tremendous loss of confidence in oneself. If the vertigo attacks occur frequently enough, there may be insufficient time between spells for vestibular compensation to occur and the person will experience chronic dysequilibrium with intermittent vertigo attacks, never having a chance to fully recover. Healthcare professionals and patients have difficulty sorting out the difference between spontaneous vertigo attacks, and the head movement or position-induced vertigo and dysequilibrium during the compensation phase.

In its early stages, Meniere's Disease can be exceedingly difficult to diagnose but early recognition and treatment may be useful in arresting the progression of the disease from its natural course of hearing and balance degeneration. Each time a hydrops (accumulation of fluid) episode occurs, it does a small amount of cumulative permanent damage to the inner ear.

Treatment for Meniere's Disease is directed toward controlling the endolymphatic fluid swelling since in 90 percent of patients no active cause will be identified. The body uses sodium as its principal regulator of fluid balance, so a strict 2000-milligram daily sodium-restricted diet is recommended. A sodium guidebook is recommended to learn about packaging labels and natural sodium content in foods. Simply removing the saltshaker from the table is inadequate to treat this disorder and strict regular adherence to a 2000 mg diet is strongly recommended while symptoms are active. Most people who do adhere to their diet notice a substantial difference when they eat out and cannot control their sodium intake, experiencing more symptoms within one or two days afterwards.

The second most important factor in controlling Meniere's is controlling stress. The hormonal release associated with stress has a profound effect on aggravating Meniere's Disease, although, the mechanism for this is poorly understood. It's quite obvious that an increase in spells occurs during times of crises, injury, or illness. Gaining emotional control over Meniere's Disease is a critical issue in preventing oneself from falling into the trap of becoming a victim to the condition. Victims live in the constant fear that an attack may occur, and the very stress of this fear actually creates more attacks. Many people who understand this situation find that they can exert their will over spells, and sometimes avert them. Caffeine, nicotine, and other powerful stimulants have also been known to aggravate Meniere's. Decaffeinated beverages and cessation of smoking are always recommended.

Physicians will often add a diuretic (water pill) to the treatment regimen to reduce the inner ear fluid pressure. Diuretics are often used for several months, and discontinued if the condition can be controlled by diet alone. If the spells cannot be adequately managed, then vestibular suppressants are often prescribed. These medications are all central nervous system depressants in nature, trying to slow down the abnormal impulses within the balance system, or anti-nausea medications that also help stabilize balance. Such medications are for symptom assistance only and do not prevent vertigo attacks. They may be used on a daily, even round-the-clock basis for short periods of time.

Medical treatment for Meniere's is generally successful in controlling the attacks, limiting them to one or two significant attacks per year, and most people don't require surgery. About 20 percent of Meniere's patients ultimately fail medical treatment and desire surgical intervention to stop the vertiginous attacks. Most of the procedures are designed to deaden the affected balance nerve so that the abnormal imbalance signals no longer reach the brain, and the vertigo attacks cease. Newer less invasive treatments are being developed but remain investigational. When there are no further disturbances in the balance system, vestibular compensation can occur as the opposite inner ear adjusts to the new balance arrangement.

7. Under what circumstances should people be concerned enough about their hearing disorder to be seen medically by a family physician, otologist or otolaryngologist?

Charles Krause, MD is Past-President of the American Academy of Otolaryngology—Head and Neck Surgery. Dr. Krause has taught internationally, has more than 100 scholarly publications to his credit, and serves on five editorial boards.

Many individuals notice a problem with their ears, and wonder whether they should see a physician before being evaluated for hearing aids. Though no guidelines are correct for every circumstance, the following situations should be reason for evaluation by an ear, nose and throat specialist (otologist or otolaryngologist). These conditions are essentially what the Food and Drug Administration recommend that your hearing care professional consider prior to fitting you with hearing aids:

a) *A visible congenital or traumatic deformity of the ear.* Many of these are accompanied by hearing loss, and most can be improved both functionally and in appearance.

b) *A history of active drainage from the ear,* particularly if it's foul smelling. Except for earwax, most drainage from an ear is caused by active infection. Left untreated, the infection can cause permanent damage.

c) *A history of sudden or rapidly progressive hearing loss.* Except when caused by a plug of earwax, a sudden loss of hearing needs careful evaluation, especially if it occurs in one ear.

d) *Acute chronic dizziness,* particularly "spinning," is caused by a problem in the inner ear, and may be associated with a hearing loss.

e) *Unilateral hearing loss of sudden or recent onset within the past ninety days.* The sooner one seeks treatment, the more hopeful the outcome.

f) *A conductive hearing loss* (air-bone gap on audiometric testing) of at least 15 dB at 500, 1000 and 2000 Hz. Such a hearing loss can usually be restored with medical treatment.

g) *Visible evidence of a plug of earwax or foreign body* in the ear canal. Such an obstruction is best removed using careful extraction rather than irrigation.

h) *Pain or discomfort in an ear.* This is usually caused by infection in the external or middle ear. Medical evaluation and treatment usually result in rapid resolution of the pain.

By applying these guidelines, you'll have a more informed idea of when a medical specialty evaluation is necessary.

8. Cochlear implants have been around now for a number of years. As an expert on this, can you tell us what a cochlear implant is, who is a candidate, and the latest achievements in this area?

William Luxford, M.D. is a physician at the House Ear Clinic in Los Angeles, and Clinical Associate Professor of Otolaryngology at the University of Southern California School of Medicine. He has been performing implant surgeries for years and is extensively published in this area.

In general, cochlear implant candidates have a bilateral severe-profound sensorineural hearing loss, receive little or no benefit from conventional hearing aids, are in good physical and mental health, and have the motivation and patience to complete a rehabilitation program. A cochlear implant is an electronic prosthetic device that is surgically placed in the inner ear, under the skin behind the ear to provide sound perception to selected severe-to-profound hearing-impaired individuals.

In addition to the internal component of the system, the cochlear implant has external parts that are worn outside the ear, including the microphone, speech processor, headpiece antenna and cable. A cochlear implant is NOT a hearing aid (see Figure 8-3). A hearing aid amplifies acoustic signals, thereby making sounds louder and clearer to the person with hearing loss. Hearing aid-amplified acoustic signals are delivered to the ear and converted into electrical impulses by hair cells of the inner ear in exactly the same manner as sounds that are transmitted to the normal hearing ear.

A cochlear implant, on the other hand, converts acoustic sound vibrations into electrical signals, which are then coded and patterned in a manner designed to enhance speech perception. Through an externally worn antenna and internally implanted receiver, these coded electrical signals are then transmitted to an electrode in the inner ear which directly stimulates the auditory nerve fibers, thus bypassing the damaged hair cells of the cochlea. The electrical impulses are delivered to the brain where they are interpreted as meaningful sounds.

Potential candidates for cochlear implants include both children and adults with a wide age range. For the most part, children are at least 12-months old, while there are many people in their 80s who are successful users. Candidates undergo a very thorough evaluation, including medical, audiological and radiological assessment. The medical evaluation includes a complete history and

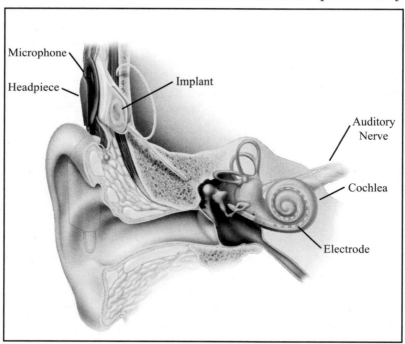

Illustration reprinted courtesy of Cochlear Ltd.

Figure 8-3: Illustration of a cochlear implant.

physical examination to detect problems that might interfere with the patient's ability to complete either the surgical or rehabilitative measures of implantation. In adults, the cause of deafness would not seem as important as its onset. Adults who become deaf later in life, and who have fully developed speech and language before losing their hearing, are able to make better use of the implant than those who are born deaf or lose their hearing very early in life. On the other hand, the prelingually deafened child, if implanted early in life, can receive a great deal of benefit from a cochlear implant.

Counseling is important so that the patient and the family will have realistic expectations regarding benefits and limitations. Support from family and friends is essential in the rehabilitative process. The definition of success is different from person to person, and family to family. Memory of sound appears to be one of the most important factors for success in adults. Early implantation, and placement in an educational program that emphasizes development of auditory skills appear to be important factors for success in children.

Initially, only those patients who were stone deaf in both ears were considered implant candidates. With significant improvements in implant technology and signal processing, the benefits gained by implanted patients, both children and adults, have markedly improved. These improvements have led to a broadening of the criteria for implant patients. Selected patients with severe hearing loss receiving some benefit from appropriately fitted hearing aids are now considered possible implant candidates. Hearing aid technology has also improved. Most likely, patients with mild and moderate hearing loss will be candidates for hearing aids. Patients with severe loss will be candidates for either a hearing aid or cochlear implant, depending upon how well they function with the appropriate device. Patients with profound hearing loss will probably receive the best benefit through the use of a cochlear implant.

9. If you could offer one important idea to readers with loss of hearing, a mechanism that would enhance their hearing ability and improve their lifestyle (in addition to hearing aids), what might that be?"

David G. Myers, Ph.D., is professor of psychology at Michigan's Hope College and the author of fifteen books, including *A Quiet World: Living with Hearing Loss* (Yale University Press, 2000).

Without hesitation I would offer to double the usefulness of their hearing aids by enabling them to serve as customized, in-the-ear loudspeakers for the broadcast of sound from PA systems, televisions, and telephones. With the mere push of a button—no hassle, no conspicuous headset—our hearing aids would broadcast phone conversation through *two* ears (all the better to hear you with, my dear!), our TV loudspeakers would be inside our ears, our public venues would broadcast sound not from speakers 40 feet from our eardrums, but from a fraction of an inch. Moreover, the sound would be customized for our own needs, by our own hearing aids.

In this dreamed-of future, doubly useful hearing aids would be more widely welcomed. With doubled usefulness—and doubled usage—the stigma of hearing loss and hearing aids would diminish. Hearing aids would come more and more to be seen as "glasses for the ears." Support for insurance and Medicaid/Medicare reimbursement for hearing aids would increase. The end result: improved quality of life for millions of people with hearing loss.

Is this an impossible dream? Actually, it's en route to becoming reality. In the UK, Scandinavia, and Australia nearly all hearing aids now come equipped with telecoils (or "audio coils," as Dr. Mark Ross suggests we rename them, to convey their broader usefulness beyond telephones) that can receive this broadcast sound. And most public venues—including virtually all churches, cathedrals, and public lecture halls that I have visited in my sojourns in Britain—have equipped themselves to broadcast directly to hearing aids (as does my own home television and office phone, through inexpensive induction loop systems).

Here in Holland, Michigan, most of our major churches and public facilities now offer hearing aid compatible assistive listening. It's common observation that the existing hearing aid incompatible assistive listening systems (transmitting signals to cumbersome receivers and then on to headsets) rarely get used. A number of churches that have switched to hearing aid compatible assistive listening are reporting a tenfold increase in assistive listening use (and who knows how many people are invisibly using this inconspicuous form of assistive listening?).

Thanks to publicity and word-of-mouth enthusiasm, hearing aid compatible assistive listening is now spreading elsewhere in west Michigan. One Grand Rapids, Michigan church sound engineer observes that, "Slowly the members of our congregation have been updating their hearing aids and (in four months) we've gone from

148

one user originally to over ten now. Several members have commented on the clarity and ease of use."

For more information on hearing aid compatible assistive listening, including where it works, how much it costs, and links to vendors, visit www.hearingloop.org.

10. Is there a problem in the United States regarding the unintentional swallowing of hearing aid batteries, and if so, what consumer protection would you recommend?

Rose Ann G. Soloway, RN, is a board-certified clinical toxicologist with the National Capitol Poison Center. She is also Associate Director of the American Association of Poison Control Centers. The National Button Battery Ingestion Hotline Telephone Number is 202-625-3333 (collect if necessary).

It's hard to imagine swallowing a hearing aid battery, but it happens more than 1,000 times each year. And it's easier than you might think. Since Toby Litovitz, M.D. established the National Button Battery Ingestion Hotline and Registry in 1982, she and the Hotline staff have managed more than 6,000 cases of battery ingestion accidents. It occurs in children and adults.

Children swallow hearing aid batteries for the same reasons they swallow other things within reach. They're curious, they explore everything within reach, and anything can end up in the mouth. They swallow batteries pried from their own hearing aids or their family member's hearing aids, or those that may be merely left on tables or in drawers. They also have been known to locate them in the trash. But hearing aids are only one source of this problem for children. They'll swallow batteries from toys, cameras, calculators, jewelry and so forth. Protection is available by using child-resistant hearing aids and by keeping batteries in their original packaging, stored out of children's reach. To dispose of batteries, wrap them securely in something before discarding, so they can't be easily retrieved.

Adults are apt to swallow batteries by mistaking them for pills. Sometimes, they're put in the same pockets as pills. People think they're swallowing pills but are later surprised to find pills, and no batteries in their pocket! A similar mistake occurs when loose batteries are stored in old pill bottles. Adults who mistakenly think they can test a battery's charge by placing it on the tongue, also wind up swallowing a tiny, slippery battery. The same thing happens to adults who put them in their mouths to keep them handy while they change batteries.

While it's unusual for swallowed batteries to cause harm, injury and death have occurred in a few cases. Most of the time, a swallowed battery passes through the esophagus and into the stomach. Gradually, it works its way through the intestinal tract and is eliminated in the stool. Rarely, the battery gets stuck in the esophagus. This situation doesn't always cause symptoms right away, but is very dangerous because it can cause a lot of bleeding. Also rarely, a battery that passes through the esophagus and stomach later gets stuck somewhere in the intestinal tract.

If someone swallows a battery, immediately call the 24-hour National Button Battery Ingestion Hotline at 202-625-3333. You may call collect. You may also call your physician or local poison center, and ask them to call the Battery Hotline. The nurses at the Hotline will ask you to have a chest x-ray immediately. If it shows that the battery has passed through the esophagus into the stomach, nothing needs to be done—or should be done—except watching and waiting for its passage. In young children, this could occur in just a day or two; in elderly people, such passage could take two or even three months. If the battery hasn't been seen within a week, another x-ray will usually be recommended to be sure it is moving. The Hotline staff will stay in touch with you until the battery has passed, then ask you to mail it in for evaluation. Of course, if you develop any symptoms, the Hotline nurses will work with your physician to decide if any treatment is necessary.

Keep in mind that it is rarely necessary for surgery to be done! Be sure to contact the Battery Hotline immediately if someone suggests surgery to remove a battery.

CHAPTER NINE

Problem-Solving and Extending the Life of Your Hearing Aids

Thayne C. Smedley, Ph.D.*
Ronald L. Schow, Ph.D. *

Dr. Smedley is currently Professor Emeritus of Audiology at Idaho State University in Pocatello. He received his Ph.D. in Audiology from Stanford. He is nationally published in areas of hearing aid satisfaction and self-assessment issues. In his many years of clinical audiological practice, he has also dispensed hearing aids. He was Chief of the Audiology Section of the Veterans Administration Medical Center in San Francisco for nine years, and also served as president of the Idaho Speech, Language and Hearing Association.

Dr. Schow, Professor of Audiology at Idaho State University, has specialized in audiological rehabilitation since earning his Doctorate from Northwestern University in 1974. He has twice been recognized at ISU with a campus-wide award as Outstanding Researcher. Dr. Schow has worked with many rehabilitation groups of hearing aid wearers, using satisfaction and other self-report questionnaires to measure successful outcomes. He's co-editor of a popular text on audiological rehabilitation now in its fourth edition.

*We both wish to acknowledge our colleague Jeff Brockett who consistently provides us with valuable input and feedback on projects like this. He has many years of experience working with hearing aid clients in a local dispensing office and in our university Veterans Administration dispensing program.

Hearing aids are electromechanical devices proven to be greatly beneficial to millions of people. Despite this fact, like any device, they are subject to breakdown. Consider that hearing aids typically are worn for long hours each day which places stress on electrical components and battery power. They exist in a relatively hostile environment of moisture, warm temperatures (especially with certain styles) and intrusive substances such as earwax, skin acids and oils. These substances may be healthy for the ear but potentially corrosive to hearing aids. Additionally, these substances can block important sound delivery pathways making the hearing aid perform poorly. For these reasons, no matter how well they're made, sooner or later they will stop working.

Hearing aid failure is almost always unpredictable and sometimes occurs at the most critical and inopportune time. Consider

Fred's plight as he headed out the door for an early meeting with upper management on his job. Fred, who had worn hearing aids for several years, was a section supervisor in a large manufacturing firm. Meetings with management occurred weekly but this one was especially important because it involved a review of company organization and possible restructuring of middle and upper management. The meeting would involve a lot of discussion which Fred needed to hear. He knew his supervisors were counting on his input. Fred was in line for a promotion and this could be a pivotal meeting for his career.

As he pulled his car out of the garage and headed down the street, he reached into his pocket for his hearing aid case, took out his hearing aids and slipped them comfortably into place. The car motor suddenly took on its normal drone as he turned the volume up. "Why is the right hearing aid sputtering?" he wondered. The aid sounded with static and seemed a bit weak. Fred arrived at work and took his place in the conference room which was already filled with 20 of his co-workers. He was just a little late that morning so he took his place in the back of the room. But he knew he would be all right as long as he could hear.

The hearing aid in his right ear continued to sputter and crackle. The company president opened the meeting and Fred's heart sank. His right hearing aid had gone dead. He hurried to throw in a fresh battery. The commotion interfered with the president's opening remarks and distracted his near-by associates; and to no avail. The hearing aid wouldn't respond. Frantically, Fred cranked up the left hearing aid to compensate. It promptly let out a wild squeal, attracting stares from his colleagues. He turned the left aid back down and sat there.

By this time, the president had finished his introductory remarks and had opened the meeting to discussion. What had the president said? Fred had caught only a small part of it and he fared no better with the other voices coming from different parts of the room. Because he was uncertain about what was being said, Fred did not feel part of the meeting. He was frustrated. He felt disappointed. He was angry.

"I hate these hearing aids!" he mumbled to himself.

It didn't help matters when his buddy George said to him on the way out, "Where were you today? I expected you to have a lot to say!"

Perhaps this episode strikes a resonate chord with you.

Hearing aid failure can be upsetting, as Fred thought it was in his case. In less critical situations, a hearing aid that quits working may only produce frustration. At the very least, hearing aid breakdown is annoying.

This chapter addresses how to keep your hearing aids performing and how to spot the cause of malfunction early when breakdowns occur. We also include tips on preventive maintenance to improve hearing instrument reliability and longevity. Remember that some hearing aid failures will be unpreventable and beyond your control. Such failure will result in "down time" on your part and may require a send-off to the factory for repair. Also addressed will be sub-par performance from hearing aids which, although working, do not function as well as they might.

But first, a few words about hearing aid styles. Some styles of hearing aids are subject to more stress and abuse than others, and the approach you should take in troubleshooting hearing aid breakdowns can vary from one style to the next. Reasons for hearing aid failure which are related to a particular hearing aid style will be noted in each section. You need to be familiar with the basic hearing aid styles of which there are five. These styles are described in terms of their location on the ear or body, and for purposes of convenience are identified by acronyms: BTE, ITE, ITC, and CIC (See Figure 6-1 in Chapter 6, page 96).

In this chapter, much of our instruction will be directed toward ITE and ITC aids because these represent the majority of styles in current use in the united States. Problems specific to CIC hearing aids will be highlighted because more and more hearing aids are being fit which are of this "deep canal" type.

As part of this introduction, a few words need to be said about hearing aid longevity. You may have asked, "How long will my hearing aids last?" Just as hearing aids will malfunction on occasion for reasons described above, it follows that they won't last indefinitely. This is true even for very expensive ones. For various reasons, cost being one of them, some wearers expect their instruments to last 10 to 15 years or more. Hearing aids that remain in useful service for this long are the exception rather than the rule. In fact, research has demonstrated that the typical hearing aid gets replaced about every five years.

Also, some hearing aids are replaced not necessarily as a result of being worn out but due to changes in a person's hearing or because individuals may desire instruments of improved technology. In any case, you're well-advised to consider five years as the average life span of most hearing aids. All things considered, proper maintenance procedures will help to extend the longevity of any given hearing aid to its optimum potential.

We present this outline of problem-solving techniques at the risk of giving you the impression that hearing aids are fragile, sensitive devices that will commonly fail and require unusual care and worry on your part. This is not at all the case. For the most part, today's hearing aids are exceptionally reliable and durable. They will serve your hearing needs day after day, year after year with rarely a breakdown.

Like your automobile, any number of problems can go wrong with a hearing aid, but for the most part, easy and relatively inexpensive remedies are available. Here are most possibilities.

Dead and Defective Batteries

The inexperienced wearer is often disappointed by what is viewed as short battery life. After all, watch batteries of approximately the same size last a year or more before replacement is necessary. Hearing aid battery life is related to two primary factors: the size (and storage capacity) of the battery and the amount of current draw required by the hearing aid. The larger the battery, the greater the storage capacity. However, the number of hours you will get from a battery depends on the current draw.

Hearing aid amplifiers simply draw heavy current loads, much heavier, for example, than those required for simple watch circuits, or even heart pacemakers for that matter. As a useful comparison, consider the common battery-operated flashlight. Interestingly, the typical flashlight uses a standard size D battery which has 1.5 volts, almost identical to the voltage of a hearing aid battery but of vastly larger size with greatly increased storage capacity. Even so, imagine how long a flashlight would work if it were used continuously for 16 hours a day as is required for hearing aids! The fact that hearing aid batteries maintain operation for long hours at a time, day after day, is quite impressive.

Furthermore, battery efficiency has improved substantially in recent years. Today's batteries will keep a hearing aid going many days longer than the older style hearing aids (for example, BB-type) whose batteries were ten times larger! Signs of a failing battery are weak output, distortion, increased tendency of hearing aid feedback,

154

intermittence and/or strange or unusual sounds such as static or fluttering (sometimes called "motorboating").

Weak and faulty batteries are a leading cause of hearing aid failure. In general, today's hearing aids require approximately 1.2 to 1.4 volts to operate properly. When a battery reaches 1.1 volts or less, the hearing aid will function poorly, if at all. The battery should then be replaced. In contrast to batteries of an earlier era, battery strength is sustained at a constant level until just a few hours before it dies, at which time it goes quickly. Older batteries used to lose power gradually over their life, requiring the wearer to adjust the volume at ever-increasingly higher levels to maintain proper output. This is not the case with today's batteries.

Anticipating the Dead Battery

So, in light of battery usage, how can you avoid hearing aid failure due to weak or dead batteries? First, you'll need to develop a replacement rhythm. Knowing the approximate time when a battery will go dead can decrease one of the sources of anxiety that may accompany hearing aid use. A replacement rhythm is most easily developed by marking a calendar each time a battery goes dead. A designation such as R-B or L-B for right aid or left aid batteries works nicely. Most hearing aids today use zinc-air batteries with a pull-tab on the back of the battery. You can just as easily stick the tab on the corresponding date on the calendar and note it as right or left replacement.

After a few weeks, you'll learn the replacement cycle required of the hearing aid and will become remarkably accurate in anticipating the impending demise of waning batteries. Calendar-marking may not be necessary after a few months, although for those with poor memory, it can be continued indefinitely.

For the technically-oriented, an inexpensive battery tester can be purchased that will read the exact voltage strength of a new or used battery. This is probably a good investment because it allows you to determine if hearing aid failure is due to the battery itself.

Getting the most out of your batteries

Today's batteries have excellent shelf life, up to one year or more if kept in a cool, dry place. (Refrigerating batteries, a common practice years ago, is unnecessary.) Most batteries used today are of the zinc-air type which means a charge does not begin until a pull-tab is removed from the face of the battery, allowing air to enter through tiny openings. Never remove the tab until the battery is to be inserted into the hearing aid.

To optimize battery longevity, disengage it when the aid is out of use for a period of time. The most common period of regular disuse for most wearers is overnight. When the aid is removed at bedtime, the easiest thing to do is simply open the battery compartment all the way and set the aid down on a dresser top or some other safe and convenient but accessible location.

Avoid storing your hearing aids on a bed table or other similar location where children and/or dogs can get to them; otherwise they're easily lost or destroyed. It's not necessary to remove the battery from its compartment. Position the aid so that the door remains open and the battery remains in it. This will simplify hearing aid start-up the next morning. Just close the battery door and the aid is ready to go. If the aid is placed on the dresser carelessly, the battery may fall out. This isn't really a problem except that it creates an unnecessary inconvenience the next morning when the hearing aid battery must be located, oriented and reinserted. For individuals with limited vision or finger dexterity, this inconvenience can be significant. If you have an aid with the "flip up" door, you will have to remove the battery in order to prevent its discharge.

Batteries in Backwards

The matter of inserting batteries, although not directly related to battery life, raises the question of another source of hearing aid failure. Batteries have a "negative" and "positive" polarity and therefore each side must be positioned correctly in the battery door to coincide with the electrical contact requirements of the circuit. The flashlight analogy cited earlier applies as well to battery orientation. We all know that a flashlight whose batteries are inserted incorrectly will not work. Manufacturers of hearing aids help with this problem as much as they can by marking a "+" sign on one side of the battery door to remind you that the positive side of the battery must be on that side. Because this "+" imprint is so small and for many impossible to see, the manufacturer also tailors the battery door to match the shape of the battery.

A close look at any battery will disclose that batteries are perfectly flat on one side (the positive side) and beveled on the other (the negative side). The battery door is similarly configured and should be studied by new wearers in its open position, under a magnifying lamp if necessary, to learn these identifying characteristics. Then you can position the battery appropriately in your fingers and insert it correctly with confidence.

Please note that with the battery in place, if the door doesn't close readily with only a minimum of force, this is often a sign the battery is in backwards. When this happens, reverse the battery and try again. In any case, *do not force the battery into place.* Doing so can damage the hearing aid. At this writing, some manufacturers are producing hearing aid circuits that will accept batteries placed in either position. This modification is in response to the difficulties some wearers have with battery insertion. This technological improvement may be the standard someday with all hearing aids.

Never insert the battery into its place by accidentally sliding it beneath the battery door. By-passing the battery door will usually not damage the hearing aid but may likely jam the battery in place and require a trip to your provider to have it removed.

As of this writing, probably about five percent of hearing aid manufacturers have implemented the use of a hearing aid battery compartment that allows you to install the battery regardless of its polarity. This is undoubtedly the wave of the future for all hearing aids, at a small additional cost. On your next hearing aid purchase, you may want to inquire about it.

Spent Batteries

Naturally, every wearer likes to get the most hours possible from every battery. To do this, some people will remove batteries that show the earliest signs of weakening and save them for later use after they've recovered some of their charge. It's true that near-spent batteries will self-rejuvenate to a degree after removal from a hearing aid and may provide power for an extra day or so. This strategy of holding onto spent batteries, however, has several problems. First, it can give you a false sense of security. Hearing aid batteries with weak voltages can fail at any moment. Secondly, and of greater concern, these batteries somehow get mixed in with the fresh batteries. The result is confusion and frustration when a bad battery is picked up and inserted in the hearing aid when it's thought to be good.

Re-using worn batteries is a poor practice because the savings is not really worth the bother. Consider the following: assume a battery lasts two weeks and costs $1.00. If you get two extra days per battery by recycling spent batteries, the result would be four extra days use per month. The daily cost of batteries using two per month at a cost of $1.00 per battery is about 6 cents ($2.00 divided by 31 days). So, four extra days at 6 cents/day is 24 cents savings per month, or less than $3.00 per year. A savings of $3.00 per year is clearly not worth the hassle of keeping track of used batteries. This also holds for binaural wearers who might save approximately $6.00 per year. Our advice is, when zinc-air batteries go dead, throw them away. Also, never leave bad batteries lying around where children can get them. Batteries can do serious damage if ingested.*

Conserving Battery Life

Some hearing aid wearers concerned with operating costs will turn their hearing aids off when they "don't need to hear." Such individuals feel they get increased longevity with this strategy, analogous to the "turn off the lights when not in use" philosophy. While there may be some justification for this practice in special circumstances (for example, while working in a noisy shop for a few hours), a habit of turning hearing aids on and off "as needed" is not recommended. You can never tell when an important auditory event will come along, such as another person's voice or a warning signal. You don't want to be inconsiderate of others by shutting off your "antenna" so you hear them only when you want to. Furthermore, it's important to be aware of the rich assortment of environmental sounds that keep us in touch with the world.

Stockpiling Fresh Batteries

With today's batteries, is there anything wrong with storing a reasonable supply? If you see a two-for-one battery special, it's tempting to take advantage of this offer and save money but we give you this caution: such "sale batteries" are sometimes promoted to get rid of old stock and might more correctly be termed "stale batteries."

If you're inclined to store a supply of batteries, our advice is to investigate the manufacture date and then purchase no more than six months' supply at a time. Beyond this period, full storage life of the batteries might be compromised. Also, you just might decide to

*Should this occur, call the National Button Battery Ingestion Hotline at (202) 625-3333 for assistance (collect if necessary).

change hearing aids before the supply is used up, resulting in an over-supply of batteries that may no longer be of the appropriate size. People who travel are well-advised to purchase an adequate supply of batteries before taking a trip, especially if traveling overseas. Try to avoid situations where you must make a purchase of unfamiliar brands which may be of poor quality or irregular size.

The Defective Battery

Present-day batteries are very reliable as a rule and you can usually depend on a fresh battery working as it should. Occasionally, however, a new battery or a whole pack will be defective. Your provider will gladly exchange them for a fresh package.

Earwax Obstruction

Another leading cause of hearing aid failure is wax blockage. The technical name for common earwax is cerumen. It's produced by a gland (actually called the ceruminous gland) in the outer ear roughly one-third of the way down the ear canal. The product of this gland is a pasty substance, usually light brown or tan in color and bitter in taste. (Take our word on this one!) Cerumen is believed to exist in the ear canal to discourage flies and insects from entering this opening.

The degree of wax generated in the canal varies greatly from one person to the next. On average, men experience more wax build-up than women. Some women, however, can produce large amounts of cerumen, as can children. For reasons not clearly understood, some individuals generate little or no wax. If you're presently unaware of the wax condition in your ears, your physician or hearing health care provider can readily inform you of this after examination with an otoscope (ear light).

Hearing aid wearers must continually be on the lookout for adverse effects of earwax. When hearing aids are inserted into the ear canals, (or earmolds in the case of BTE hearing aids), they can slide alongside or directly into accumulated wax. The fresher the wax, the softer and more easily it can get pushed into the sound bore (receiver) of an aid. A thin smear of earwax over the receiver (sound) tube will shut the aid down instantly.

Preventing Wax Build-up

The first defense against wax build-up is regular cleaning of your ear canals by a physician or audiologist, or as simply as it sounds, in a shower by direct spray into the canals. The cautions here are to be careful of the water pressure, and be certain you don't have a hole in the eardrum, or any other condition which might prevent such easy management of earwax.

Hearing instrument specialists are generally not trained to remove earwax, and while wax removal is within the scope of practice for audiologists, many prefer not to provide this servce. In any case, you are well-advised to locate a person or office that will provide this service as needed. Attempting to control build-up of earwax by regular use of cotton swabs is not recommended. Aside from the possibility of doing physical damage to the ear canal or drum (the "don't put anything in your ear smaller than your elbow" concept), cotton swabs will usually only serve to pack the wax deeper with each attempt. By looking into the ear, professionals can readily discern the cotton swab users, as the wax shows a nicely formed concave surface down in the ear canal.

Some hearing aid wearers with chronic wax problems may find regular use of "ear lavage" effective. Equipment along with instructions for home use are available in many hearing care offices and drug stores. Wax softeners for use prior to cleaning can also be purchased. Some people may be uncomfortable squirting water into the ear canal. A discussion with your physician would be advisable before attempting it. The main problem with this type of treatment is the difficulty knowing when the wax is all out.

The second defense against wax blockage is utilization of some type of wax guard. There are a number of commercially available products which suit this purpose. Many manufacturers now provide such a device as original equipment. Directly, or under magnification, you can look into the sound opening of the hearing aid to see if a wax guard is there. These common devices include "spring," "Band-Aid" or "trap-door" style guards. All such devices should be discussed with your hearing health care provider who can explain service requirements.

Responsibility for Wax Maintenance

This is not to say that whoever dispensed your hearing aids has primary responsibility to keep them free of earwax. You need to develop a daily habit of inspecting the end of the hearing aid where the sound comes out and looking for wax blockage. If accumulation is noticed, this wax can be readily removed in most cases.

When and How to Remove Wax

The best time to inspect hearing aids for wax is at the close of the day. At this time, any accumulated wax will still be soft and more easily removed. If you use the Band-Aid style guard, you can wipe across it gently. After a few days if you observe the cushion separating from the adhesive backing, remove it altogether and replace. If used properly, you'll never need to clean out the receiver (loud speaker) which is the rubber housing hole at the tip of an aid.

If your hearing aids have the wire coil in them, you may use a device known as a wax loop. This is merely a wire looped around the end of a piece of plastic. Gently insert it into the receiver tube, turn it one full rotation, then remove. Avoid picking or poking. Clean any debris from the loop. Nightly cleaning has the added advantage of keeping the receiver tube open for more adequate ventilation and drying. Review this procedure carefully and thoroughly with your provider so that inadvertently you don't damage your hearing aids by cramming the wax loop into the wrong opening (such as the microphone port on the face of the hearing aid) or too deeply into the receiver port which can damage the speaker diaphragm.

Additionally, a wax tool that is a little too large to fit readily into the receiver tube can push the tube itself down into the shell of the hearing aid. This will damage the instrument, often causing it to squeal, resulting in needed repairs.

Wax should also be removed from hearing aid vents. This is the other port in the hearing aid next to the receiver (loud speaker) port. It can be identified because vents are longer, they do not have a rubber housing through the channel, and often run the length of the earpiece or earmold. This also means they're not as easily cleaned. Some people have resorted to the use of wires of various gauges to ream out vents. Wire should be used with caution as it can crack the shell. Large vents are less likely to get plugged up and much easier to clean. Pipe cleaners work extremely well for large vents, such as ITEs, and light gauge fishing line for vents in CICs. Your provider will have suggestions for obtaining these and other suitable tools for cleaning.

Sometimes, wax build-up becomes dry and flaky before it's

removed. When this happens, a good brushing of the hearing aid openings can be helpful in addition to use of the wire loop. When brushing, always hold the hearing aid upside down so that wax particles fall out of, rather than down into, the hearing aid. Also, keep your brush clean so that wax particles which collect in the bristles from previous brushing aren't injected inadvertently into the openings.

Ear Discomfort

Like pressure on the feet from a tight fitting pair of new shoes, hearing aids can occasionally be uncomfortable. Unlike feet, however, such discomfort in the ear is not tolerated well. Hearing aid-related ear pain can distract from intended amplification. Discomfort associated with hearing aid use usually has a specific anatomical site of origin but a widespread reaction. That is, a tight-fitting earmold may cause specific tenderness in one spot in the ear canal but in time the sensation can radiate. Additionally, accumulation of earwax and moisture may result in periodic ear discomfort.

Causes of Ear Discomfort

The most common cause of ear discomfort is an ill-fitting earmold (in the case of BTE) or hearing aid shell (in the case of ITE, ITC or CIC). Earpieces are fabricated from impressions taken of your ear. Usually they'll fit precisely. They're designed to fit snugly but not uncomfortably. It should be realized, however, that your degree of hearing loss will have a bearing on the tightness. Severe hearing losses must have a tight fit to prevent feedback (whistling).

There are two causes for ear discomfort which can result from a poorly fitting hearing aid or earmold. Either the earpiece was made improperly or incorrectly positioned in the ear. Impressions can and usually do provide exact replicas of the ear canal. This is because most providers are experienced in taking ear impressions. Occasionally, however, impressions can be distorted during preparation, while in transit to the laboratory, or during fabrication.

Another factor affecting comfort has to do with jaw movement. In some cases ear pain is caused or aggravated by movement of the jaw when earpieces are in place. For many, movement of the jaw can have significant influence on the shape of the canal. This is really quite normal. The effects of jaw movement can be felt by placing the "pinkie" finger deep in the ear canal while moving the jaw. (Try it while you're reading this). This movement arises from the joint of the lower jaw called, technically, the temporomandibular joint, or simply TMJ.

Even though earmolds may have reflected accurate impressions of the canal, the resulting earpieces may not "give" when the jaw and ear canal are moving, as when talking or chewing. If you suspect a poorly fitting earmold or hearing aid due to influences of the TMJ, you may want to discuss this matter with your hearing care professional.

The second most common cause of ear discomfort is the earpiece which is placed incorrectly in the ear. Figure 9-1 shows both proper and improper insertion. Earmolds that have been accurately fabricated can cause ear pain if not inserted correctly. When placing the earmold or hearing aid in the ear, you must make certain the device is "seated" into its exact position or it can create pressure points in the canal. Difficulties with correct placement is a common problem, especially for new wearers.

Those who use BTE hearing aids, for example, must make sure the entire earmold is properly placed. A common problem here is when the earmold is inserted into the canal, the uppermost portionisn't tucked into the groove of skin at the top of the ear. This incomplete placement can shift the angle of the earmold just enough to create a tender spot down in the canal. ITE wearers can have the same problem.

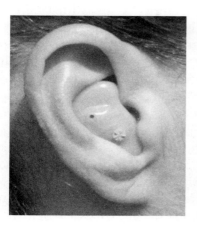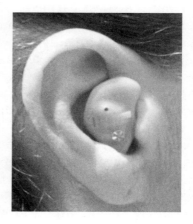

Figure 9-1 The *correct* (left) and *incorrect* (right) placement of a shell-type hearing aid in the ear.

Those who try CIC instruments may experience some fitting and placement problems initially. The deeper a hearing aid is placed in the canal, the more sensitive the canal tissue. Some wearers are simply reluctant to push an aid fully into the canal, fearful that doing so will cause pain. This is understandable. Also, there can be concern the aid can be pushed too deeply into the canal and cause damage. This also is a logical concern. However, ear canals tend to be carrot-shaped (that is, the deeper into the canal, the narrower the opening) and the aid cannot be pushed without discomfort beyond its appropriate location.

With practice, however, you will soon get a "feel" for the exact location of the aid and should be able to insert it correctly with confidence and without discomfort. If the hearing aids are difficult to insert, repeated "fiddling" can also cause discomfort. Special earmold lubricant is available to assist in the insertion. If placement difficulties aren't easily resolved, practicing proper insertion of the hearing aid in the presence and under the watchful eye of your provider is helpful and reassuring.

Correcting a Fitting Problem

Ear discomfort associated with a new set of hearing aids can be either transitory or persistent. If you're a new wearer, you should understand that initial discomfort of a slight degree can be expected. Normally, we wear nothing inside the ear canal, so tolerating that first earpiece will require some adjustment. Such discomfort will subside substantially or be completely gone after only a few days. Again, it's like adjustment to new shoes.

Discomfort which persists after going through an initial adjustment period is another matter. Unrelenting discomfort present each time the hearing aid is worn should certainly be noted in follow-up visits with your clinical audiologist or hearing instrument specialist. During such visits your provider will either need to modify the earpiece by grinding or buffing, or remake the fitting by taking a new impression. It's helpful here to note that in most situations of poor fit, satisfactory corrections can be made right in the office. Also, please be aware that most wearers don't experience these initial difficulties at all and "hit the ground running" with new hearing aids. Often, we hear in our office, "I forget they're even in my ears!"

Plugged Up Vents

A vent in an earmold or hearing aid is simply an open passageway or tube that extends from the front of the earpiece to the tip. It almost always exits the tip very close to the sound opening (receiver tube). Except in the case of more significant hearing loss, a vent will always be present. The diameter of the vent may be either large or small. In general, hearing aids fit to people with mild loss will have large vents while those fit to individuals with more severe losses will have smaller vents. They're usually placed in earmolds or hearing aid shells by manufacturers. They can also be placed there or modified by your provider. Vents should always be kept open to perform their intended function.

Purposes for Vents

Vents are placed in earpieces for four rather important reasons. They allow sounds that you may hear normally to enter the ear canal directly without being amplified. You don't want to block the ear to sounds which you hear normally. Vents that serve this purpose are usually fairly large and obvious. This type of vent is very helpful if your hearing loss affects only higher pitches (technically called frequencies).

The second purpose of venting is to reduce amplification of unwanted sounds. Often these are low-pitched tones which you may already hear normally. Experienced, and sometimes even new wearers will report hearing better when their provider enlarges the vent by drilling. This diminishes low-pitch bothersome background sounds. Hearing aids and earmolds fit to those with more severe loss will require smaller vents.

A third purpose of venting, perhaps the most important in some fittings, is to decrease the acoustic effects of your own voice. You'll readily identify this as the objectionable sounds of your own voice while the ears are blocked off. This is called the "occlusion effect," as described in the previous chapter. It's the "my voice sounds like I'm talking in a barrel" effect.

Moisture Problems

Handling moisture problems will depend on what type of hearing aids you own. The use of water to remove wax or dirt from any part of the hearing aid itself is inadvisable. Moisture is a natural enemy to electronic devices. The use of a dry cloth or tissue to wipe clean the *outside* surface of the hearing aid is the only recommended cleaning practice.

With regard to BTE style hearing aids, earmolds used with these instruments must be removed from the hearing aids before cleaning. They can be soaked in a solution of soap and warm water, gently scrubbed clean, then completely dried before re-connecting to the hearing aid. Two methods we recommend for drying is a hand-held, forced-air blower which simply pumps air through the tubing, or a can of compressed air (typically used to blow dust off computer keyboards). Failure to dry earmolds will risk moisture seepage into the aid.

Another useful tool in keeping moisture from being a problem is regular use of a dehumidifier. Comercial versions are available and very reasonable. The device is simply a container for your hearing aid with a built-in, moisture-absorbing chemical. The hearing aids are placed in the container anytime they're not being worn. The device aborbs accumulated moisture and leaves the hearing aids dry. The chemical eventually becomes saturated with moisture but can be recharged by heating it in a warm oven. Be sure to follow the manufacturer's instructions.

As noted earlier, ear canals can produce a degree of moisture which can affect hearing aid performance. Like the problem of earwax, the amount of moisture present in human ear canals can vary widely from person to person. Your activity level and climatic conditions in which hearing aids are worn are two of the more common variables affecting moisture build-up. People with high levels of physical activity who perspire easily can be more prone to moisture problems than those who lead a more sedentary life.

Moreover, a moisture problem can be further aggravated by conditions of high humidity. Moisture build-up can result from either internal or external sources. Internal sources are those related to the condition of the auditory canal while the latter refers to liquids which arise from outside the ear, as those, for example, associated with rain or severe perspiration.

The Effects of Moisture

While BTE-type hearing aids, if maintained properly, can outlast in-the-shell types, they tend to have the worst problem with moisture. Water vapors arising from the canal condense in the connecting tube. When these vapors reach a region outside the canal of slightly cooler temperature, condensation converts to small droplets of water which appear as tiny bubbles in the tube. The accumulation of enough water droplets can be sufficient to close the tube and shutdown amplification.

Externally-produced moisture surprisingly is less of a problem. Rain water, unless very severe or persistent, usually runs around the ear and off the head with little or no adverse affects. A worse condition, especially for BTE use, exists for the person who perspires a lot. With such individuals, beads of perspiration form in the hair along the top of the hearing aid. In time, this moisture can seep into the cracks and openings along the upper surface of the hearing aid and eventually affect operation. The case of the postal worker comes to mind whose daily walking route involved extreme outside weather conditions. The operation of his BTE hearing aid was little affected by rain water which was easily diverted by wearing a wide-brimmed hat. Heavy perspiration, however, caused predictable shutdowns during workdays of extreme heat and high humidity. It's worth noting here that proper care and maintenance will reduce mechanical problems associated with moisture.

Hearing aids of the type worn in the ear have less difficulty with moisture build-up. Externally produced moisture with in-the-shell-type hearing aids tends to flow around rather than into the ear as a rule. Also, the further the aid is placed inside the canal, the less the problem as moisture from the canal lining has less of an opportunity to get into the receiver tube. Therefore, CIC's are the least affected by internal and external moisture.

Resolving Moisture Problems

The point was emphasized earlier that moisture and electronic devices are a poor mix. To every extent possible, moisture in the region of the ear must be avoided. This means, to state the obvious, that hearing aids are not to be worn while showering, bathing, or swimming. They should also be removed before getting into a hot-tub, steam room, or while participating in water sports of any kind. These precautions apply equally well to moisture-related exposures such as spray paint, spray deodorant, hair sprays, and most aerosols. Chemicals in these particles are particularly destructive because they leave permanent residues which build up over time. With repeated use, they are certain to cause eventual hearing aid failure and permanent damage.

When hearing aids are unavoidably exposed to moisture, as with individuals who must work outdoors, extra precautions must be used. In the case of the postal worker cited earlier, a simple plastic sleeve slipped over each BTE instrument resolved the problem without significantly affecting performance. Some hearing aids are constructed specifically with watertight gaskets and are more weatherproof than others. Actually, most recent vintage hearing aids are surprisingly resistant to water damage and function in a variety of situations without intermittence, especially if they can thoroughly dry out overnight.

In this regard, hearing aids should be left in the open air when stored overnight with battery doors open, especially if moisture build-up is a problem. The use of dry-packs which absorb moisture can also be used to advantage during storage. These dry-packs are inexpensive and available from your hearing care professional.

Other drying techniques may also be tried. One recent BTE wearer who had a chronic problem with moisture solved it by dangling his hearing aids (overnight) *upside down* by the earmolds from a homemade wire hanger. In this position, moisture was more readily able to escape from the hearing aids than when they were stored laying flat which tended to trap the moisture.

It should be noted that hearing aid failure due to moisture is not always easy to diagnose. Except for water vapor forming in the tube of BTE hearing aids which is readily visible, moisture is difficult to observe. If hearing aid stoppage is found to be unrelated to the more obvious causes, such as faulty batteries or wax blockage, then moisture build-up should be suspected. The use of drying procedures previously described should help isolate this problem. Also, perhaps with the help of your provider, you could check your daily routine. For example, it will do little good to faithfully dry out hearing aids overnight if every morning after they're inserted you apply a healthy portion of hair spray!

Short Battery Life

Shortened battery life will result most likely from one of three possibilities: the battery is defective and has a weakened charge; the hearing aid is defective and draws current in excess of what it should;

or the battery routinely is left in operation in the hearing aid during periods of disuse (for example, overnight). Wearers who are always careful to disconnect the battery overnight can usually assume a defective aid in the situation of poor battery life. While batteries can be faulty on occasion, as noted earlier, most commonly it will be the hearing aid itself at fault. When this happens, the likely solution is factory repair.

Before an aid is returned to your provider with this problem, it's wise to verify that your present batteries in use are in fact good. Because battery life can vary somewhat within acceptable limits, we recommend taking action with the hearing aid only when battery life is consistently one-half of what it regularly has been or should be. This would help to confirm a defective hearing aid. Otherwise, you might be dealing simply with variability in longevity among batteries.

The Problems of Intermittence

We have touched upon a variety of hearing aid problems to this point, each of which can cause some degree of intermittence: a bad battery, a fleck of earwax, a little moisture. In addition, hearing aids can develop intermittence from other causes though these may be less frequent.

Dirty Volume Control

Hearing aids that still use volume controls (some current hearing aids don't) operate on the basis of metal contact points that slide against each other in normal operation. You can almost feel movement in the contacts as you rotate the volume wheel up and down. These contact points can become corroded with dirt or other residue that will not allow current to pass. This may occur when the volume control is in certain positions where corrosion is the worst. The result is an aid that goes on and off or even produces a very audible static noise as it's being adjusted. If you experience this problem, we recommend you rotate the volume control knob in continuous movements back and forth between low and high power up to 20-30 times. If this does not resolve the problem, it will require factory cleaning and/or repair.

Dirty Battery Contacts

Battery contact points can also become corroded and create similar problems. As with the volume control, dust, moisture, and earwax are the primary culprits. Corroded contacts in the battery compartment result in intermittent or stopped current flow which has a direct effect on hearing aid output. Corroded battery contacts are also quite difficult for you to clean and will require office or factory servicing.

The Problem of Oily Skin

Some individuals with oily skin have battery contact problems. During routine handling and insertion of batteries, oily residue can be transferred from finger tips to the surfaces of the battery and adversely affect contact pickup. Such oily film can cause intermittence. If you suspect this problem, replace batteries with an ordinary tissue to prevent their surface "contamination," or be careful to wash your hands thoroughly before handling them.

Overview

It should be noted in summary that during regular use, it's impossible to prevent a certain amount of contamination of hearing aids from elements in the environment. Sooner or later these elements are bound to affect instrument performance. The auto mechanic, for example, who works in a greasy, dust-laden environment is highly susceptible to hearing aid corrosion. Intermittence and frequent servicing should be expected when hearing aids are used in such unfavorable environments.

Intermittent problems can be difficult to diagnose. One strategy is to rule-out the most obvious causes. Often, when a hearing aid quits working, the first thing that comes to mind is that the battery is dead. An easy test is to take the battery from the other side (assuming it is working) and place it in the hearing aid that is not working. If the hearing aid begins working, then the problem was the battery and a new one can be activated. If it does not work, then other problems, such as wax build up, battery contacts, etc. may be to blame. Similarly, a battery in question can be placed in the working hearing aid to see if it has adequate capacity.

Poor Telephone Reception

If hearing and understanding speech are difficult face to face, even with hearing aids, then telephone reception will be similarly difficult. Likewise, if your hearing aids allow you to function well in a face to face situation, you should converse with little difficulty on the telephone.

At the outset, it should be noted that some people have no difficulty hearing on the telephone without their hearing aid. This is because the telephone system has some built-in amplification, and a telephone held closely to the ear can provide adequate pickup while blocking out some background interference. Individuals with greater loss will need additional amplification to hear well on the telephone. On the other hand, those with severe to profound loss may be unable to converse at all on the telephone, with or without amplification. To explore what telephone amplifying devices are available to you, see Appendix I.

Whether you use hearing aids or not for the telephone, if you're in the presence of noise, cover the mouthpiece each time after you speak. This prevents undesirable room noise from traveling into your telephone receiver and being amplified into your own ear (or hearing aid), adding confusion to what you may already be finding difficult to hear.

The Telecoil Circuit

One mechanism developed to improve telephone reception that has been available for many years is the telecoil (short for telephone coil). Not all hearing aids have them. If yours has it, you'll see some designation or switch on the case. BTE-type hearing aids with this device will have a switch position labeled "T." In-the-shell hearing aids may simply have a manual two-way switch. Because the telecoil circuit requires extra space, smaller hearing instruments such as the ITC or especially CIC will not have them.

Telecoil circuits work by processing electromagnetic waves produced by the telephone receiver (a process known in electronics as induction). When the hearing aid switch is on "T," a special wire coil is activated within the hearing aid circuit in place of the microphone. The only sounds that will come through the hearing aid in this position is what you hear through the telephone. Background noise near the telephone, for example, is unamplified which is a big advantage. Hearing aids with T-coils (as they're called) should work on nearly all currently available telephones. Telecoils can be quite satisfactory for mild to moderate hearing losses.

Successful Use of the Telecoil Circuit

Review of your Operator's Manual will familiarize you with the telephone setting. If the hand-switch on the aid is not set to the telephone mode, only the regular microphone will pick up sound which may provide inadequate reception. To get the best reception from the telecoil, the receiver of the telephone must be positioned within the most sensitive area of the hearing aid. To find this position, simply move the telephone earpiece around the ear during conversation until the voice comes in loudest. Your provider will be more than happy to demonstrate this procedure on an office telephone.

Other Tips for Improved Telephone Listening

Selection of the most appropriate hearing device is the first step toward successful telephone use. The clinical audiologist or hearing instrument specialist should be consulted during the selection process so that your individual needs are given full consideration. For some, telephone use is of little consequence. To others, it may be critical. For this latter group all possible telephone options need to be carefully explored.

The next most important step is practice. Optimum telephone pickup is often achieved only after periods of trial and error. When asked about telephone use, an occasional hearing aid wearer will say, "I tried it once but it didn't work." You'll need more patience than that. Don't expect to get your best results after only one or two attempts. Practice is especially important here and the best way to get practice is to prearrange a long telephone conversation with a friend or relative. Explain that you're experimenting over the telephone with your new hearing aids. A patient listener will allow you to try your hearing aid in a variety of telephone positions (or perhaps hearing aid settings as well) until you achieve optimum reception. Such practice will result in success with the telephone in a wide majority of cases. Also realize that poor telephone reception can be the fault of the telephone in isolated cases.

Hearing Aid Squeal (Acoustic Feedback)

Feedback is the term we use for the high-pitched squeal commonly associated with amplifiers which have microphones and loudspeakers connected to them. This is the case with hearing aids (see Chapter 6, page 98). The squeal is caused by amplified sound that radiates from the speaker, is inadvertently picked up by the microphone and gets continuously re-amplified. The same thing can happen in an auditorium when the loudspeaker and microphone are too close together, or the amplifier volume is set too high. The hearing aid is said to "go into oscillation," and the squealing sound coming from the loudspeaker is the result. Feedback can be avoided when the sound coming out the loudspeaker is prevented from reaching the microphone.

In the case of hearing aids, the pathway of sound from the loudspeaker opening (receiver) to the microphone input is along the side of the hearing aid or earmold in the ear canal, or through a vent. If the earmold or shell-type hearing aid fit snugly into the ear, and the vent is not too large, sound is unable to leak out and reach the microphone located outside the ear canal, in which case the aid won't squeal. When hearing aids or earmolds fit too loosely in the canal, the opposite can result. In general, a loose-fitting hearing aid or earmold is more likely to squeal than a tight one. Also, a high-powered hearing aid will have a greater tendency to feedback than a low-powered aid and therefore will require a tighter fitting earmold. Competent hearing care professionals realize that the size and placement of hearing aid vents must be determined with the utmost regard to the potential for feedback.

Acceptable Versus Unacceptable Feedback

We want to emphasize that acoustic feedback is a natural phenomenon of amplifiers and not of concern, in and of itself. Feedback is to be expected, for example, when a hearing aid is "on" and held in a cupped hand. It does no damage to use feedback in this way to tell if the hearing aid is working. Similarly, it's usually not a problem to purposely cup the hand to the ear and listen for the "beep" as the hand is moved toward and away from the ear. Many wearers test the hearing aid in this way to be sure it's on. Others will rotate the volume control to the position of feedback during adjustment. Here again, this is no problem. These are all examples of predictable and acceptable feedback.

Unacceptable feedback is the type that spontaneously rings without warning or provocation, that happens, for example, while you're chewing, brushing your hair, scratching the side of your head, or tilting your head downward. This latter movement causes a slight shift in the position of the hearing aid, sometimes just enough to allow sound to leak out. The squeal associated with all of these activities can be vexing. Feedback of the unacceptable kind also occurs when you try to turn the volume of the hearing aid up to a more desirable level but cannot because the aid starts to squeal. At this volume position, with you attempting to extract the last decibel of sound possible, the aid is on the verge of feedback and will squeal at the least little disturbance. These are examples of feedback which you will not want to tolerate. Almost all of them can be corrected.

Earwax and Feedback

Feedback can occur anytime sound is deflected toward the microphone. Normal eardrums tend to absorb energy so that if an earpiece is reasonably snug, leakage is minimal and feedback doesn't occur. Earwax, on the other hand, seems to absorb very little sound and will bounce the sound right back out of the canal toward the microphone. Therefore, individuals who experience unexplained feedback should have their ears checked for wax build-up.

Solving the Feedback Problem

People with the most severe hearing loss provide the greatest challenge to their provider when it comes to feedback control. Most of it is still manageable. As noted earlier, a first consideration in dealing with feedback is to ensure that your ear canals are clear of wax. This does not usually require a medical evaluation each time the ears need to be checked. The audiologist or hearing instrument specialist can do the job just as well and usually at no cost. If the canals are obstructed, your provider may charge a fee to remove wax, or if necessary refer you to a physician. You may want to insist that examination of your ear canals be a part of regular office hearing aid check-ups.

Given clear canals, the next obvious concern in dealing with feedback is the fit of the hearing aids. The most common cause of all feedback problems is poorly fitting earpieces. Sometimes the hearing aid or earmold are ill-fitting from the very beginning. Hearing aids that have been used for several years without a feedback problem can gradually develop it as the aid "loosens up" in the ear. This results from two possibilities. If you wear BTE's with earmolds, the earmolds can shrink and change shape. Also, tissues along the wall of the canal can gradually give way to small but persistent pressure associated with the instrument—the shoe and foot analogy again. This problem of increasing tendency for feedback is pronounced in children whose bodies undergo relatively rapid changes. Therefore, more frequent remakes can be expected with this age group to control feedback, especially in cases of severe loss.

Feedback with New Purchases

If you have purchased new hearing aids that squeal or act like they're always on the verge of squealing, or do when volume is moved up to a desired level, insist on getting the problem corrected— the sooner the better. Correcting a feedback problem with a new fitting is most easily done during the initial issuance.

Some feedback problems can be corrected readily in the office while the more severe cases may require a remake of the fitting. This will involve, of course, taking new impressions and going without the hearing aid for a brief time. But the temporary inconvenience will be well worth it. Whatever you do, don't allow the problem to go uncorrected, thinking, "Well, in time it'll probably straighten itself out." A feedback problem will rarely go away on its own. If anything, it usually gets worse. Left unattended, a feedback problem can result in a fitting that is less than optimal.

Feedback and Telephone Use

Feedback occurs most often when some object is placed next to the hearing aid. This object can be a telephone, your own hand or even a nearby wall or other flat surface. Feedback is not a problem with hearing aids (having a telecoil circuit) when the switch is in the "T" position. However, it is a common problem with non-digital hearing aids. Digital hearing aids have feedback managing capabiltiies.

With analog hearing aids, careful positioning of the telephone receiver by moving it a slight distance from the ear or tilting it at a slight angle often eliminates feedback and still allows adequate reception. Some hearing aids are less susceptible to feedback than others. CIC-type instruments, for example, are the most feedback-free. If feedback is a problem for you, a donut-shaped, sponge-like product that fits onto the receiver of the phone can be purchased from your provider or ordered directly through a catalog from one of the companies represented in Appendix I.

Static and Other Unwanted Sounds

Be assured that unless you happen to be listening to an old radio badly tuned to the station, internally generated static of any kind is abnormal and in need of correction. Static resulting from internal causes means that the noise is created from some problem inside the hearing aid or telephone and not existing in the environment.

Recall that for the hearing aid to have clear sound, adequate battery voltage must be maintained. Likewise, current drawn from the battery must be appropriate or the hearing aid can produce strange sounds. In cases of low voltage or dirty contacts, cleaning or replacing the battery, or servicing the contact points in the battery door should correct the problem. Moisture and dirt in the volume control or other switches can also cause static. Here again, cleaning and regular servicing will help.

Sometimes strange sounds including static-type noise come through the hearing aid even though it's relatively clean and the batteries are fresh. This can be caused by defective components in the amplifier. These components can wear out in time and require replacement. Also, some hearing aids will pick up strange sounds that radiate from electrical appliances or light fixtures, especially fluorescent. Such sounds are externally generated. Hearing aids that pick up these kinds of unwanted sounds seem to be less of a problem now than with older hearing aids. Regardless, if you detect a problem that you think may be caused by such a thing, bring this to the attention of your hearing care practitioner to solve.

Another source of unexplained sound coming through a hearing aid that should be mentioned here are those sounds in the environment that you may have forgotten existed or you've not heard for a long time. New wearers often pick up on these *new noises* right away. One such person complained, "Since I bought these hearing aids, I hear a terrible noise in my kitchen I never heard before. It's mostly constant but sometimes it goes off for awhile. What's wrong with these hearing aids?" A courtesy home visit revealed that what she was hearing was the compressor of her old refrigerator! Obviously, she hadn't heard this noise for a long time. Other sounds to which you'll need to become re-acclimated are common noises associated with motion, like paper rattling, water running, utensils dropping on a plate, and wind.

Wind Noise

If you spend a lot of time outdoors, wind noise can be especially bothersome. If so, you might want to investigate a CIC-style fitting which will eliminate or greatly reduce wind sounds. For non-CIC instruments, a "windhood" or "windscreen" can be installed that can also help the problem. Discuss these options with your provider.

Background Noise

The single largest complaint of hearing aid wearers is difficulty hearing in the presence of background noise. Unfortunately, hearing aids, even the most expensive ones, have difficulty separating the sounds and voices you want to hear from those in which you have no interest. So you'll have to learn to put up with a certain amount of noise just as people with normal hearing do. The new programmable hearing aids do offer some relief for those who must function regularly in noisy situations.

Preventive Hearing Aid Maintenance

Few consumer purchases have any faster rate of depreciation and limited resale value than hearing aids. Stated differently, from an economic standpoint your hearing aids are of no value to anyone but you. For this reason and because they're expensive to replace, it makes good sense to service them on a regular basis. Systematic maintenance will reduce repair costs, lessen the number of "down" times, and most importantly extend the life of your hearing instruments. What follows is a brief list of maintenance procedures that will help you to accomplish this:

- **Clean Your Hearing Aids Daily:** This is best accomplished by first wiping the hearing aids with a dry cloth or tissue to remove wax, oil and moisture from the surface. Then lightly dry-brush all components using the wax removal techniques described earlier, and remove wax from the receiver and vent tubes. This cleaning should be done daily, preferably at bedtime.
- **Proper Storage:** Place hearing aids in a safe, convenient

and protected location, being certain to disengage the battery door in a manner recommended previously. Sticking hearing aids in pockets or at the bottom of purses without a protective container exposes them to dirt and dust that can eventually do damage. Dust-free carrying cases are provided with nearly all new hearing aids. You should have this case available when necessary. If moisture build-up is a concern, store the hearing aids in a closed container with an absorbent dry-pack available from your provider.

- **Schedule Regular and Periodic Checkups with Your Provider:** In-office cleaning and servicing are usually included free with your purchase of hearing aids and you should take advantage of this. We recommend servicing be done at least every three months (like servicing an expensive car). Hearing aids should be checked for power loss, dirty contact points, plugged vents and openings, and so forth. A more comprehensive servicing should be performed at least annually. This should include electroacoustic analysis (test box evaluation to ensure maintenance of original manufacturer's performance specifications). BTE wearers should also have the tubing replaced at this time (if not needed at 6 months). There may be a modest charge for this more comprehensive servicing but it's worth it. Residents of drier climates like Arizona will need more frequent tubing changes than those living in more moist environments like Louisiana. Next to daily cleaning, regular in-office servicing is the most important maintenance you can obtain.

Have a Spare Set of Hearing Aids

We conclude with a discussion of hearing aid spares. We hope it's clear from the information contained in this chapter that basic knowledge of hearing aid operation together with use of simple maintenance techniques can go a long way to preventing hearing aid breakdown. We hope it's also apparent that despite your best efforts, without warning, your hearing aids can fail from time to time. If you're a person who's totally dependent on your hearing aids in order to communicate, you might want to consider the purchase of backup hearing aids for use in emergencies. Maintaining two sets of hearing aids may initially cost more. It could be argued, however, that two sets used more or less alternately will last twice as long as one set used full time.

So, spare aids may not cost more in the long run. It's like the wisdom of owning two pairs of shoes versus only one pair. For some wearers, this works. Also, the availability of spare hearing aids removes the anxiety that might accompany this loss. Some dispensers provide loaner instruments which may or may not be suitable to your personal needs but is worth inquiring.

How can you judge whether you should have spare hearing aids? The best test we know is an honest answer to the following question: *Does the mere thought of even a temporary loss of the use of your hearing aids create in you the slightest tinge of anxiety?* If it does, then you probably should have a spare set.

Actually, the availability of "spares" is something we all insist upon with commonly used devices we consider vital. (Our cars have spare tires, for example, so we can avoid panicking when a tire fails.) In our experience, people with severe hearing loss will regularly maintain a backup set of hearing aids, especially when the livelihood of such individuals is dependent on good hearing. Furthermore, the federal government for decades has issued to eligible military veterans two complete sets of hearing aids so that good hearing won't be interrupted by temporary breakdowns. You may be one who would also like the extra security of backup instruments in case yours go in for repair.

Backup hearing aids can be the still-functioning old set that you just replaced with new ones, or where money is of lesser concern, they can be hearing aids of more current vintage. If you choose to purchase or otherwise have available a set of spare hearing aids, try to ensure that they take the same size battery as your regular ones. This will lend itself to far more convenience than having to store and maintain two different kinds of fresh batteries.

Hearing Aid Disuse and Longevity

The question arises, "Will my spare hearing aids wear out faster or maybe even slower if they're not used regularly?" It's true that peak performance of electromechanical devices can decline with disuse. This need not happen with spare hearing aids, however. This is avoided by rotating them periodically with your regular instruments, for example, once each month or more. This level of activity will keep them running and assure you that they're available and working if and when needed. During extended periods of storage

(30 days or longer) the batteries should be completely removed so as to prevent corrosion from possible leakage. While cost is a serious consideration, two sets of hearing aids is ideal.

Help From Family and Friends

Sometimes you just need a little help. Your spouse, family member or friend can provide that help with problem solving. As hearing aids have gotten smaller, so have the batteries. Sometimes the batteries are difficult to insert and remove from the hearing aid. Having someone help you orient the battery so that you get it in right will avoid the consequences of getting it in wrong and possibly damaging your hearing aid.

Inserting and removing your hearing aid can be difficult and if the hearing aid is placed in your ear improperly it may not function properly or even irritate your ear. A family member or spouse can help you make sure that the hearing aid is fitting correctly and well positioned in the ear.

The openings in your hearing aid where sound is delivered to your ear are very small and when they become blocked with debris this will keep you from hearing at your best. Sometimes, the cleaning process requires small tools and it can be a frustrating process when you have difficulty seeing. A friend or family member can help with the cleaning to make sure your hearing aid is working properly.

Probably the best help you can get from a friend or family member is their help in monitoring your communication ability. You may not always be aware of communication that you are missing or problems with the hearing aid. This person can alert you that your hearing aid is making that "squealing" from feedback or an adjustment is needed in order to hear better. Friends and family can help out with just about every aspect of problem-solving and extending the life of your hearing aids.

Conclusions

Today's hearing aids, products of an unprecedented technology, are creations of remarkable quality. Their more accommodating size, improved performance overall and generally high reliability are characteristics as impressive to most audiologists and hearing instrument specialists as they perhaps are to you. They're built to operate for long hours under adverse conditions and they do so with batteries that, while smaller, work harder and produce more energy for their size than those of an earlier era. For the most part, these hearing instruments perform their valuable service unfailingly.

CHAPTER TEN
Aging and Hearing Loss
James F. Maurer, Ph.D.

Dr. Maurer received his Doctoral Degree in Audiology from the University of Oregon Medical School in 1968. In 1971, he developed and directed the first mobile auditory testing and rehabilitation program in the United States for low-income older persons, which carried on for more than two decades. He has written and co-authored seven books and many articles on hearing loss and aging. His efforts in Costa Rica establishing an Audiology diagnostic testing clinic, which bears his name, earned him a Governor's Commendation. He was also instrumental in the discovery of a new hereditary deafness syndrome. Dr. Maurer is a Professor Emeritus at Portland State University in Oregon.

This chapter is dedicated to you with hearing loss who have passed the fifth decade of life. It's also written for friends and family members who desire to understand the personal consequences of auditory loss in older persons. There is much within this chapter aimed at teaching rehabilitation strategies for helping yourself and others, so that both of your lives are enriched by the experience.

I don't mean to be a snob, but I'm not a great believer in growing old. Having passed the big "Seven Ohhh," I think I can now understand why some people get face lifts, dye their hair, lie about their age, fall for quick fix rejuvenation supplements and even, like my dear mother, disassociate from others of the same age because they "look even older."

Not that I have acquiesced to any of these strategies, you understand. But I did experience a secret moment of exhilaration a few days ago when the lady in the pro shop made me pull out my I.D when I asked for senior golf rates. And I admit to avoiding the kid who sacks groceries at the checkout stand because he once offered to carry them for me. In fact, if he even looks at me I quickly shove two fingers through the plastic bag loops, lift them off the counter like they're weightless, and try not to sway like a drunken sailor as I exit.

So whatever it takes to make you feel young and viable is okay. It's like one of my hearing-impaired oldsters said to me when I was a wee lad of forty-five. "You don't quit playing the game because you've grown old. You grow old because you've quit playing the game."

181

He wore his hearing instruments constantly.

As stated earlier in this book, among the great chronic health conditions of the sixty-five and older group, hearing impairment ranks *number three,* right after arthritis and hypertension. While it might seem we are dealing with a minor epidemic, the truth is we start losing our hearing very early in life.

Most experts now agree that age-related changes that affect our hearing are in the inner ear, the auditory nerve, the brain stem, or the auditory part of the brain. It is interesting to note that most changes due exclusively to aging don't present a whole lot of hearing problems. In fact, there are many older persons who can put up with a few misunderstood conversations and neither they nor their friends perceive loss of hearing sensitivity as a problem. These people are fortunate. Fully a third of 50-plus persons in the United States have real impairments. Over age seventy, the incidence of hearing impairment increases to nearly 50 percent. But this is not entirely due to growing old.

Many of us not only have a touch of presbycusis, but we've picked up a few other causes of hearing loss on our trek through life. We also undergo a gradual depletion of cells in the auditory processing part of our central nervous system. Once these neurons within the brain stem and brain structures are depleted, they're not replaced, although we now know that nature compensates for dead cells by establishing new connections around them. Moreover, scientists recently have discovered ways of preventing neuron destruction. In fact, some neurons have been "rescued" even after damage had already begun!

Changes due to aging at this "central" level don't show up in a conventional hearing test, yet they do account for many aging issues. There's reduced short-term memory span. There's lengthened reaction time to auditory signals. Try keeping up with your grandkids playing an arcade game! As we age, we may experience difficulty tracking a fast-paced conversation or shifting gears to a new topic.

Lucky for us Walter Winchell was doing his "rapid fire" commentary when we were kids! We now find ourselves having more difficulty understanding speech, especially in background noise and particularly the "noise" of other people talking, such as in a cafeteria.

A 61-year-old woman confided in me that she was seated in a beauty salon, trying to read a new diet book. Finally, in a moment of exasperation, she put it down. "I simply couldn't concentrate with all those people talking! I never used to be this way."

Even in a fairly quiet place there's a greater problem paying attention ("Great sermon wasn't it?"). The drone of sounds that become neural noise may be someone speaking, or the neighbor's lawnmower, or music playing. Even our thoughts at the moment can interfere with our ability to concentrate on something else, causing us to make poor judgments or creating a momentary lapse of memory, such as when driving a car ("Honey, you just missed our exit!"). We simply cannot handle as many inputs as we used to, and it's harder to focus on what we're doing when there are multiple hearing challenges.

Sometimes changes associated with aging can be misinterpreted as hearing impairment. An older couple came into my office for a second opinion. Urged by her husband, the woman had purchased two hearing aids, which she was wearing with some discomfort. Upon examining her I found that her hearing was normal for her age, sixty-four years, she had excellent word discrimination. After testing her ability to repeat sentences presented in cafeteria noise, I found she had a slight, but not clinically significant difficulty. In this instance, the husband's perception of his wife's "hearing impairment" was incorrect.

What additional testing revealed was a problem with short-term memory. Her husband would ask her to bring something from another room, and she would interrupt her activities in the kitchen to do what he asked. Then she forgot what it was that he wanted. He took this to mean that she didn't hear him, which was not so. She had simply forgotten. We older folks can identify with this short quip titled, "Enigma:" *Where did I put what I saw before it went?*

Psychologists have known for years that aging affects our ability to recall things in the immediate past more than our ability to remember the distant past with our "crystallized" intelligence. Does this mean we get dumber as we age? No. Does it mean we aging persons have trouble with a task that requires *new* learning? No, but our minds may not be as nimble as they used to be. Does it mean we're more likely to forget someone's name after just being introduced than a playmate's name recalled from childhood? Yes! Is this a new problem for us? No. We've forgotten things stored in short-term memory all our lives because we were distracted or focused on something close, or simply forgot. This is not "new" behavior. It's just that as we grow older, it increases in frequency, often because of neural noise interference.

Living with a Hearing Loss

Even a slight hearing impairment during this time of life may occasionally affect our ability to understand others. Since the voices of people with whom we talk vary in those characteristics that contribute to understanding, we misinterpret some individuals more than others. Voices differ in pitch, loudness, quality and output (words per minute), each of which can influence the clarity and intelligibility of the speaker's voice. Words spoken are more understandable for some voices than others. The clearer speaking person utters words that are more precisely formed, or articulated.

Obviously, teenagers can keep up with the accelerated speech of their age group. But many of us cannot. We simply have to ask them to speak more slowly.

Broadcaster "hype" has turned "hyper" for many of us who remember all too well the comfortably paced, resonant and clear voices of the golden age of radio. Today, radio and television stations that still endorse clear and reasonably paced communication are not as easy to find. Since some voices are clearer than others, it pays to shop around the networks and public broadcasting for better listening experiences.

Visual cues, seeing the speaker as she or he is communicating, contribute to our getting the message. But constraints in our communication environments differ considerably. Some places are worse than others, where messages spoken reverberate from bare walls and floors and are lost in the wake of their own noise. In rooms containing carpets and drapes that are farther away from outside traffic noise, interference is minimized. Something to think about if you're apartment shopping.

Places where older people congregate should be stellar listening environments. Unfortunately, this is not always the case. I recall visiting a dozen or more senior adult centers, noting the fact that while most were clean and pleasant, many were located in high noise areas and few attempts had been made to reduce interior noise. One center was actually located under a roller skating rink!

If you're reading this because you have an older parent or grandparent with hearing problems, keep in mind that it's much easier to converse with them in a quiet room. Make sure there's good lighting and try to maintain a speaking distance of less than nine feet. You'll be pleasantly surprised at how much easier conversation becomes and how much stress is reduced.

Background sounds around us can also be a positive experience. We constantly monitor the world we live in, often unconsciously. Our hearing sense, as well as our vision, keeps tabs on what is happening in our space. There's often comfort in the constant background of sounds and sights in our environment. There's a sense of belonging.

Even a very mild hearing loss can change this monitoring behavior and affect how we feel. As one 56-year-old woman described to me before she began wearing hearing instruments, "Not being able to hear little background sounds was an experience I wouldn't like to repeat. I had entered an upstairs art gallery in an old community college building. Normally I would expect to hear hushed conversations, feet shuffling or other sounds. Except for the clack of my shoes on the old wooden floor, there was complete silence! I must have been the only one in the gallery, and I began to feel anxious. It was as if I was the last person alive on this planet. I hurriedly left the place...and I didn't even know why."

Like brush strokes on a canvas, the myriad of small sounds that we're so accustomed to hearing tell us we are a part of reality. They also contribute to our sense of security. Detection of some warning signals may be challenged by our hearing loss, sounds such as footsteps on carpet, tires on soft snow, or even fire burning in the next room, as one hapless 77-year-old apartment dweller recounted to me. He had barely escaped from the burning building.

Hearing loss dampens the enjoyment of some activities that gave us pleasure in the past: theater-going, music appreciation, church services, watching television, dining out, having a drink in places with background noise, talking to others on the telephone. Even a mild hearing loss can reduce life satisfaction for some things we once took for granted.

There is an acoustic issue that afflicts a few of us. We are all blessed with tiny tubes that extend from the back wall of the throat (behind the nose) into the middle ear cavities of each ear. The purpose of these Eustachian tubes is to ventilate the middle ears with fresh air. The tiny mouth of each tube is normally closed, but may open when we yawn, cough, or snore, thus permitting air to come in. Now comes the rub.

The mouth of the aging tube may tend to remain open in some cases. This condition is not something to get excited about, but for some persons it creates the complaint, "My voice echoes." And sometimes when they wear hearing instruments that amplify their voices, they say, "My voice echoes a bit louder." So an open Eustachian tube can cause voice echo, and wearing a hearing instrument may make this echo a little bit louder. Some people are troubled by this and some are not. Hearing care practitioners are experienced in helping those who are uncomfortable with this condition.

None of us are alike. We differ because of genetic influences, environmental effects, and luck of the draw from injuries and diseases that damage us permanently. The specific problems that we encounter with our hearing deficit also differ, as do our physical and emotional capabilities to overcome adversity, lifestyle, support system of friends and relatives, tolerance for breakdowns in communication, the severity of our hearing impairment, and whether we have successfully pursued professional help. What we have in common is that we will circumvent a lot of future problems by seeking quality professional help in getting evaluated and discovering the resources available to us.

Other Influences that Affect Hearing

The amount of loss that we accrue in growing older can be compounded by the consequence of exposures to other events or agents that damage our hearing mechanisms from infancy onward. These include noise exposure, diseases, high fever, head injury, toxic chemicals and drugs, blood supply deficiency, lack of oxygen and genetic influences.

Some of these causes are preventable, such as further damaging our ears from noise exposure. Some are not, such as familial or genetic loss of hearing, although microbiologists are getting closer to a solution to even this problem. In any case, it's rare to find a hearing loss that is not impacted by non-aging causes, especially among men. Noise exposure is a most common cause of reduced hearing sensitivity. According to the National Institute of Deafness and Communication Disorders, more than 30 million Americans are exposed to hazardous sound levels on a regular basis. Of the 28 million Americans who have hearing loss, about one-third can attribute their hearing loss, at least in part, to noise exposure. Older persons are no exception. Because many of us pursue noisy hobbies in later years, the topic bears further discussion.

While the Occupational Safety and Health Administration (OSHA) has required noisy industries to provide ear protection since 1970, this partial solution came too late for many who are now retirement age. We live in an industrialized society where noise is seemingly omnipresent. We were endowed with eyelids to keep out most light while sleeping but no "earlids" to suppress background sounds of traffic, air conditioners, furnaces, and a host of other noise sources that are pervasive in our homes. In fact, we are indeed fortunate if we can sit in the quiet security of the living room, close our eyes, and hear nothing.

Both community and recreational noise has increased over the years with the rise in population and proliferation of noisy vehicles and gadgets. Intrusion by other people's noises in formerly quiet neighborhoods often taxes our patience and our hearing ability. Automobile boom boxes, chain saws, lawnmowers, firearms, noisy vehicles and 50-plus years of Fourths of July all have a cumulative effect.

Other places include jazzercise facilities, which often feature loud music, and where the more vulnerable ears of infants parked in strollers in the back of the room are unprotected from this clamor. Beauty salons can be very noisy, but fortunately some manufacturers of hair dryers are now building quieter machines.

Older men often spend time in home workshops, where electric drills, saws, sanders and other equipment can add to the hearing loss associated with aging. The intrusion of jet sleds, all-terrain vehicles, snowmobiles, high volume music in unwelcome places, such as parks and wilderness areas add to mental confusion and the physical demise of delicate inner ear structures. Shooting high-powered rifles, magnum pistols and shotguns is a very efficient way to lose decibels of hearing as well. In fact, conventional ear protectors do not completely protect against such firearms. And usually we don't even know our loss of hearing sensitivity is happening until it's too late for it to recover.

Women who are homemakers are not immune to this onslaught. Some years ago my graduate students did a sound level survey door-to-door, interviewing women and measuring the noise intensity of home appliances to which they were regularly exposed. Guess what took First Place honors, the loudest ruckus of the week:

an ordinary vacuum cleaner generated a whopping 105 decibels at one lady's ear. By OSHA standards, she was running the risk of permanent hearing damage by operating that machine more than one hour a day!

Neither presbycusis nor noise-induced hearing loss is medically correctable. But they can combine to produce a greater hearing impairment. We can't turn the clock back and start wearing ear protectors at an earlier age, but there's something to be said for protecting what hearing we have left. I carry an inexpensive pair of foam earplugs for use on long airplane trips and other situations where noise exposures may be loud or lengthy.

I find it interesting, having provided hearing tests on a number of rock musicians back in the early 1970s, that many who were slow in requesting advice on hearing protectors now seek advice on hearing instruments. I wonder about the hearing sensitivity of their audiences, the baby boomers, who are now joining our aging population. Our children and grandchildren seem to perpetuate the thirst for loud music, despite our warnings and presentiments.

Adjusting to Hearing Loss

Do you remember when someone first called you "Sir" or "Madam"? Did you experience a momentary flicker of surprise, an evaporating thought that you somehow must be different from that moment on? It was as if you had suddenly arrived on some plateau in life from which there was no return.

Interestingly, our arrival may have more to do with our biological age (how old we look and feel) than our chronological age (how many birthdays we've celebrated). Some of us look our age, some of us don't. Realization of our hearing difficulties can be like that, when someone younger gives us the bad news, "Dad, you've got to do something about your hearing!" We are different from that moment on. However, for many of us there's no sudden realization. Since our loss of hearing sensitivity is usually gradual, it may take us a long time to recognize that we're having increasing difficulties associated with the loss.

An older gentleman living in a townhouse called this to my attention. "We used to hear the clock ticking," he said.

"What concerns me," his wife added, "is that we don't hear the gas jet in the fireplace anymore."

It's also interesting that some rather important sounds in our lives disappear without a whimper. A 74-year-old gentleman insisted that his new hearing instrument had a strange noise in it. He kept cocking his head and saying, "There it is again." Then he handed the aid to me. I listened to the instrument and shook my head. "I don't hear any noise, except normal background sounds."

He put the instrument back in his ear, listening, and he could hear it again. His face lit up when we both realized he was hearing his breathing for the first time in years.

Hearing old sounds again is like visiting old friends. It's a very positive experience. Some of us don't accept hearing loss so readily. And this lack of acceptance creates a quandary for the specialist trying to help us.

John was a 70-year-old longshoreman who came to my office announcing that his physician told him he had the arteries of a 30-year-old. He flexed his triceps and asked me to feel them. "Hard as steel," I responded, knowing what was coming next.

"Doc," he shouted, "I don't have any trouble hearing. I don't know why they sent me here. I can hear a pin drop."

But he couldn't. In fact, he couldn't hear a brick drop. Not only that, he couldn't understand conversational level speech. And ability to hear in noise? Forget it!

I always have great compassion for such patients. I know they want to stay young. They want to have youthful hearing skills. They don't want to wear hearing instruments because they see them as another indication that their bodies are growing older. But not tending to the needs of our ears is like letting a garden go to weeds. Tiny hair cells and nerve cells in our hearing mechanism depend on sound stimulation. Not wearing hearing aids is a poorer choice.

Another reason why denial takes place is manifested by the slope of the hearing loss on the audiogram (see Chapter 3). When we look at our hearing test, most of us see a hearing sensitivity curve that drops off—getting poorer in the high frequencies. We may still hear low-pitched sounds very well, but we don't hear higher-pitched sounds. Thus, telling this person, "You're not hearing!" is not entirely true. Some sounds may be heard quite well. Others may not be heard at all. Nevertheless, our ever-active brain fills in the blanks, sometimes correctly, sometimes not.

Grandpa and his grandson Joey were painting the shed. Joey said, "Gramps, let's go get some **thinner**."

Grandpa laughed and shook his head incredulously. "**Dinner?**

Why son, we just had lunch!"

This illustrates the difference between <u>hearing</u> and <u>understanding</u>. Joey's grandfather *thought* he heard the message. In fact, he correctly heard five out of six words spoken by his grandson. But he didn't hear one critical consonant, the soft /th/ sound, so his brain tried to fill in the blank. This small misperception changed the entire meaning of his grandson's request. When this starts happening to us frequently in conversations with others, we're overdue for help!

Many of us endure the typical high frequency hearing loss that Grandpa experiences. Such a loss allows us to hear the louder vocalized speech sounds, as the /a/ in the word ba*ll*, but we have trouble with the softer and higher frequency consonant sounds in words such as **th**igh. These voiceless consonant sounds, like /F/ in the word *F*ish and /S/ in *S*ee, contribute much more to our understanding of human communication than do voiced sounds like vowels and voiced consonants. Not hearing the voiceless sounds because of the slope of our audiogram creates errors for us in interpreting messages, even though we hear the lower frequency sounds quite well—perhaps even normally. So, we may reject the fact that we have a hearing impairment simply because we hear *some* sounds well. Such a paradigm leads to the remark, "I can hear you, but I can't understand what you're saying."

The high frequency loss may create a quandary for us when we *see* a bird singing, but don't *hear* its song, or when someone draws our attention to the chirping of crickets, the whisper of wind in the trees, or the swishing of clothing. Missing a sound also can be an unnecessary annoyance.

A gentleman in his fifties told me, "I couldn't understand why every time we went to the cabin I ended up with more mosquito bites than the rest of the family. Then one time my daughter pointed out that there was one buzzing around my ear. I realized suddenly that I hadn't even heard it!"

I used to routinely advise people with hearing instruments to take them off before going to bed. One 82-year-old woman was offended by that statement as a cardinal rule. "I've slept on my left side and worn one hearing aid in my right ear for over ten years," she admonished. "Who knows who might be knocking on my door in the middle of the night? Or what if the phone rings? I might miss something!"

A few indomitable individuals take immediate and aggressive action to counteract a recently discovered hearing difficulty. One gentleman bounced into my clinic like a bandy rooster one morning, gesturing wildly and shouting, "How do I get some hearing devices?"

When I asked him why he thought he needed them, he said that he no longer could understand his patent attorneys at board meetings. "I have to depend on what they say. Trouble is they mumble separately. If they all mumbled together," he quipped, "I think I'd understand what they were talking about." He wanted a quick solution, and he wasn't about to let a hearing impairment stand in his way. This was a man who was used to making adjustments. He was 82 years old. Did I say "old?" I mean *young!*

Others of us refuse to accept our impairments as we do our chronological age, by ignoring senior citizen discounts in restaurants and malls, because of the embarrassment in admitting the truth. Similarly, we may ignore the pleas of others by not appearing in hearing clinics willingly. Often, our late appearance is a begrudging one, something we're doing for "them," but not for ourselves. Some even deny that they want to hear. "Look, I can hear most things around me," a 57-year-old attorney said, folding his arms. "There's a whole lot going on out there that I don't want to hear. I hear just fine!"

His wife sat quietly in the corner, realizing her husband included her in what he did not want to hear.

Often our reluctance to seek help presents a barrier to those attempting to talk with us. If straining to hear is fatiguing, imagine what it must be like for another person who has to keep repeating all day.

The denial of aging is often projected as a stigma against hearing instruments that are for "older" persons. This can become an attitudinal disclaimer that hearing difficulty is not an important part of our lives. A glass of water won't suffice when we're thirsting for the Fountain of Youth. Some of us even engineer our lives to convince ourselves that we hear normally. We simply minimize our exposure to situations where the hearing deficit compromises our enjoyment of life!

I asked a woman in her late fifties, "What things did you do ten years ago that gave you a lot of satisfaction?"

She responded, "Let's see, I was very active in the church. I really enjoyed that. I taught Sunday school. I went to a symphony about once a month. Oh, and bridge club. That meant a lot to me ten years ago."

"Are you still enjoying these activities?"

She was quiet for a moment. "Well no, not really," she shrugged. "It became too much work teaching those children, and too much fussing to get ready for the symphony. I moved onto other things, I guess."

As we talked on, it became clear that she had sacrificed part of her life satisfaction because of increasing hearing difficulties. She had carefully limited her activities so that the impairment wouldn't affect her life. And she had accomplished this without ever admitting that the cause of her withdrawal was her inability to hear. Fortunately, this woman turned out to be an excellent candidate for aural rehabilitation, where she was involved in group counseling. Once she could identify with other women in the group who had similar problems, her self-esteem increased and she began to move out of her self-imposed isolation.

Because there are situations where we honestly feel we can hear normally, in front of a blasting television, for example, it becomes easy to blame others for our social inadequacy. In the hearing health care field, many of us have heard the following during an interview with an older couple.

"<u>He</u> doesn't hear what I'm saying."

"<u>She</u> doesn't speak up!"

When you think about it, we all project our problems onto other people or other things at some point in our lives. How many times have we heard statements like, "I know where I got this miserable cold—that sneezing kid in the shopping mall," or, "You forgot to remind me that I had a meeting!"

There's nothing unique about a hearing-impaired person projecting his or her problem. We all need a scapegoat at times, in order to reduce our stress. Similarly, we may find withdrawal appropriate for some situations, such as a frustrating conversation in a noisy room. These ways of avoiding or escaping from stress, denying the problem, compensating for it, projecting it, withdrawing from it actually make us feel better when our backs are against the wall. They help us maintain a positive self-image, which takes a beating when we can't hear well. But if carried too far, these bailout behaviors can interfere with getting help and reducing our life satisfaction.

Compromising our lives in order to convince ourselves that we hear normally is an all-too-common experience among those of us with impairments. Like the woman described earlier, curtailing formerly enjoyable activities can seriously reduce enjoyment of life!

If you find you're no longer showing up at holiday parties, club activities, homes of friends or other previously reinforcing events, take a good look at yourself. Maybe it's time to seek professional help.

What's also missing here is social responsibility. We hearing-impaired people owe others the right to conversations that are free of frustration. We owe our friends freedom from continually having to repeat conversations. We owe them an honest appraisal of our hearing difficulties.

What is not realized by many of us is that once we can hear better, we may discover a rebirth of more youthful participation in social activities. We become better social companions. As one wife exclaimed, "When he puts those digital instruments on, he's more like himself."

Retiring Comfortably with a Hearing Loss

It's interesting to talk to people with auditory problems who have recently retired. Some experience a sudden loss of power, the ingratiating experience of sliding backwards down the slope that leads to non-person status in the eyes of once admiring co-workers. Normal hearing people may experience the same thing. This was the feeling that a recently retired physician related to me. His repeated returns to his beloved medical school, where he had held an office for more than thirty years, were met with disengaging smiles and chafing comments like, "What are you doing back here?"

He began questioning whether a prejudice was operating because of his new hearing instruments, his whiter-than-others' hair, and the fact that he was retired. Ultimately, he felt that his once respected opinion no longer mattered, and with some reluctance, he ended his visits.

Some years later after my own retirement, he called me. "You know," he said, "if you ever write another book or have to counsel a lonely retiree, you might remember this piece of advice: if you live alone and your world is passing you by, be grateful for what you have left. Then make yourself important to someone. You'll be pleasantly surprised how important you become to yourself."

He was embarking on his third trip to China to help children with birth defects. He had decided that nothing could get in the way of his need to help others, neither hearing aids, aging body, nor unresponsive colleagues.

We are a diverse population, we older persons. Some of us cross over to retirement more slowly, tenaciously clinging to our previous roles in life through occasional work or social and service activities. We may express joy at having left our working selves behind. We network with friends seeking a newfound freedom, finding companionship in the excitement of long-awaited travel, new recreational activities, educational pursuits, or greater involvement in hobbies. Some of us don't retire at all.

Hearing loss does not respect our differences. We find individuals with auditory difficulties in all lifestyles. What's important is that we don't let this problem curtail our pleasures in life. A pharmacist friend who had been a trap shooter since boyhood was left with a significant high frequency hearing impairment in both ears. He wears two hearing instruments in retirement, and when I visit his home I always take a handful of earplugs. He constructed a woodworking shop in his garage and now creates quality furniture both as a hobby and to supplement his pension.

He and his wife are very happy in retirement, and I was prompted to ask him, "If you had it to do over, would you give up thirty years of shooting?"

"No, I wouldn't give that up. Nor these either," he grinned, pointing to his ears.

Enjoyment is found in a quiescent lifestyle for many of us. Our activities may be limited to television viewing, reading, eating, sleeping, and occasionally making visits to friends, relatives, church, and senior adult centers. We find pleasure where we can and enjoy predictability in our lives.

One such individual, age 72, has neuropathy in his hands. Because of this lack of feeling, he can no longer operate his hearing instruments. He has been perfectly content with his adjustment to his impairment because his lifestyle does not involve a great number of social activities. He's an avid sports fan, and enjoys watching these contests vicariously.

One of his concessions to his hearing difficulty is a pair of earphones connected to an infrared television amplifying system. This "assistive listening device" is easy to manipulate. It allows him to turn up baseball games as loud as he wants without interfering with adjoining apartment tenants. He also has a telephone amplifier. Such devices (as described in Appendix I) are very useful in supplementing or substituting for traditional hearing instruments.

Regaining life satisfaction may mean letting go of some of our former attitudes about aging and hearing loss and beginning to accept the realities of a new emerging self. It helps to take stock of all the positive attributes in our lives. There are people who like us for who we are, wrinkles and all. They could care less about our need for prosthetic devices. They care about us. They accept our baggage. In fact, it becomes so much a part of us that the people we care about don't even see it anymore.

It also helps to look around at the place where we spend most of our waking hours. What are the positive attributes in our home environment? What things produce pleasure for us? If we close our eyes, how many of these things would no longer be pleasurable, such as a picture that is dear to us, or a good book? If you could close your ears and hear nothing, what things of enjoyment would be missed?

Now take inventory of positive activities outside the home, things we like to do with our time. This could include hobbies, meetings, entertainment, and activities that are more physical, such as walking, fishing, travel, golf. If we apply the same limitations to our activities, in turn, closing our eyes and ears, what would the effect be? What enjoyable activities would we have to give up?

What we discover from this simple exercise is that first, there are many positive things operating in each of our lives. Getting older is not a virus that takes away all our satisfaction with life. Second, recounting our pleasures with one of our senses "closed" eliminates many positive aspects of our lives that we would not give up willingly.

Now hang onto that thought, because not giving up is exactly the attitude that must persist if we are to realize our most positive potential in spite of our hearing loss. This means accepting ourselves wearing devices that will open up a part of the world's pleasures that would otherwise be forsaken. It means accepting our new selves.

Interestingly, the world will accommodate our new self-image, and we can now move forward with our lives. People began to like us better because we are *real* in projecting who we are, and we're happier for that experience. Popeye probably said it best, "I am what I am, and that's what I am!" Did he wear hearing aids? You mean you didn't notice?

During the aging process, we consciously or unconsciously make other adjustments as well. Our eyes admit less light than in former years, so we try to adjust our reading habits accordingly, or reduce some activities such as night driving. Ability to understand conversations in background noise becomes diminished, so we try to avoid the incompatible combination of noisy places and conversations.

We find quieter places to converse. Knowledge of reduced physical stability makes us move more cautiously in risky situations where we might fall, such as walking down steps, getting into the bathtub, climbing a ladder. We discover that sudden movements can produce dizziness or unsteadiness, so we avoid quick changes in position. Diets may change to cope with various health conditions after age fifty. We find ourselves getting less sleep at night because of awakenings, and may discover a decrease in the quality of sleep. So we may compensate with naps. And the list goes on.

Compensating for perceived changes is a healthy, friendly way of insuring survival and happiness. It is taking charge of one's life. It's making a positive statement about the aging years! Like the old adage that a graying dowager told me years ago, "There may be snow on the roof, but there's fire in the furnace!" And stoking that furnace, managing one's life experiences, reducing the impact of a hearing difficulty by acknowledging the problem to others, getting professional help, and arranging living places so we can hear better, are giant steps in the right direction.

Helping Yourself

Arranging where we reside, eat, work, play or pray means getting closer to the source of sound, i.e., TV set, stereo, church pew, or the waitress in a cafe. What we're accomplishing by favorably positioning ourselves in living situations is improvement in understanding communication. The greater the distance we are from the sound source, the more distortion we'll experience, whether we realize it or not. Besides, there are those visual cues: facial expressions, mouth movements, gestures, and body language. These nuances of visual communication may not be visible from a distance but do help to actually clarify the message up close.

Stage-managing our lives also means getting away from distracting or overpowering noise or loud music. One may enjoy the power of organ music and sit close to it in a place of worship, but at what cost to hearing the message? If one ear is better than the other, favor the "good" ear. Think of places in your life where it's difficult to hear: sitting in the back seat of an automobile, sitting in a breakfast nook adjacent to the humming of appliances, standing at the cash register in a busy restaurant, or before the agent in a bus terminal. Make a list of these noisy places in your life and then think of alternatives.

196

Reluctance to get help actually may stem from any of several factors, many of which surfaced in a survey we once conducted among several thousand low income older persons. Cost of hearing appliances ranked number one. Fino et al,[1] reported on a general population study which indicated that older persons with hearing loss who did not buy amplification said hearing instruments were too conspicuous, too expensive, too noisy, and drew attention to the impairment, in that order.

Dr. Kochkin[2] cited admission of a hearing loss made people look old and disabled. Vanity (how we perceive our appearance) was also a prevalent reason. Many of us still find wearing eyeglasses more "fashionable" than hearing aids. Perceived geographic isolation from clinics providing hearing instruments ranked high on the survey, as well as lack of mobility. Older folks tend to view other health problems as more serious than their hearing impairment, despite the fact that it can degrade their mental health. My thought to those in the 50-plus age group who have hearing difficulties is that there are ample reasons for finding out what gains these instruments now offer. We may lose more by not helping ourselves if we fail to try them.

Helping a Loved One in a Restricted Environment

If you know someone in a nursing home is benefiting from hearing instruments, keep tabs on their ability to use them. Does this person have the skills and dexterity to put the instruments in the ear, turn them up, and remove them before going to bed? Can the individual change the batteries when appropriate? Is the family physician checking to see that the ear canals are free of wax buildup? Does the nursing staff complain of hearing aid whistling? This "feedback" can be caused by earwax. Is someone remembering to open up the battery doors at night, saving on battery life during sleeping hours?

And while we're at it, is anybody cleaning this person's glasses once in a while? Remember, visual skills also help the hearing-impaired person. If your loved one can no longer manage prosthetic devices, ask who in the nursing staff is responsible. In many cases I've witnessed, the primary person who cares and oversees the maintenance of your loved one's prosthetic devices is you!

Strange things happen to hearing aids in nursing homes. They can be stolen, substituted for someone else's instrument down the hall, uncomfortably stuck in the wrong ear, chewed on or digested by someone's visiting dog or cat, dropped in the toilet, plugged with wax, sentenced to lifetime solitary confinement in a dresser drawer, stepped on by a 250 pound attendant, or awaiting invitation under the bed to the fraternal order of dust bunnies.

If the instrument seems to be helping the older person only by making him or her more alert, take this as a positive sign and reward the use of hearing aids. If you make a visit and find it's not being worn, check to make sure the aids are working. It's wise of you to participate in getting the hearing aids in the ears during your visit. Chances are your warm gestures of touching, smiling, talking and caring will have positive consequences on this special person. And on you, as well.

You may be reading this book to find out what you can do for a loved one who sadly can no longer understand the printed word, cannot write effectively, or may be wandering in that personal void associated with severe mental deterioration. Unfortunately, the lower the level of intellectual functioning, the poorer the prognosis for gaining much benefit from amplification. But check first to see if increasing the volume of the soothing sound of your voice seems to create a pleasant experience, or even an increase in understanding.

I took some graduate students to a nursing home to do hearing testing on some residents. One gentleman sat very quietly in a corner of the hallway not socializing with anyone. He just looked emptily at the opposite wall. One of the staff told us he had been diagnosed aphasic, which is lack of speech understanding and expression due to brain damage. We had brought with us a powerful body hearing aid with a big red volume control. We placed it in a harness on his body, hooked his right ear up to it, and slowly began turning up the volume. His mouth opened slightly, his head turned toward us, and as we watched, a wisp of a smile turned into a full-fledged grin. One student tried to subdue her excitement and quietly asked, "Can you hear me?"

He looked at her, lips moving, eyes glistening, and managed an "uh...Yes!" A few weeks later, after we had showed him how to use the aid and charge the battery each night, I returned to see how he was doing. I found him sitting on the sun porch, holding hands with an elderly woman, talking quietly. The big box with the red volume control hung like an Olympic medallion on his chest.

References

1. Fino MS, Bess FH, Lichtenstein MJ, and Logan SA. Factors differentiating elderly hearing aid users and nonusers, <u>Hearing Instruments</u>, 43, 2.6, 8-10, 1992.
2. Kochkin S. Why 20 million in U.S don't use hearing aids for their hearing loss. <u>The Hearing Journal</u> 46(4):36-37, 1993.

CHAPTER ELEVEN
Improving Your Listening and Hearing Skills
Mark Ross, Ph.D.

Dr. Ross received his doctorate at Stanford University. He has worked as a clinical audiologist, a director of a school for the deaf, Director of Research and Training at the League for the Hard of Hearing, and as a professor of audiology at the University of Connecticut where he's now Professor Emeritus of audiology. Currently, Dr. Ross is an associate at the Rehabilitation Engineering Resource Center (RERC) at the Lexington Center in Jackson Heights, N.Y. Among his activities for the RERC, he writes a bimonthly feature on Developments in Research and Technology for *Hearing Loss: the Journal of Self Help for Hard of Hearing People.*

I don't know any hard of hearing person who, if a magic wand could be used to wave away his or her hearing loss, would not jump at this miraculous opportunity. I know that I would like to be at the head of the line! But life is not a fairy tale and magic wands are in short supply. For most of us with hearing loss, it's simply a pain, one whose impact we're constantly trying to overcome or minimize. We don't approach the world as "hard of hearing" people, seeking acceptance as a separate social entity.

On the contrary, we're trying not to make it a defining condition of our personal identity by striving to reduce the impact of hearing loss in our lives. To realize our goal of continued engagement with the larger society—with our friends, family, jobs, and interests— we employ the modern technology of hearing aids and other assistive devices. And we use various communication strategies to reduce the inevitable consequences of hearing loss.

By "communication strategies" I mean any activities that might increase your ability to understand speech, either generally or in particular situations—not just technological solutions. Of course technology is vitally important, but the adjustment process doesn't end there. There are other things you can do to improve your ability to communicate in different situations. When you purchase hearing instruments, you depend upon the hearing healthcare provider's expertise to help in making the proper decision. When it comes to communication strategies and making the best use of all types of hearing technology, *you* have to take the major responsibility. The concept of personal responsibility for one's own action underlies the three recurring themes stressed throughout this chapter: acknowledgment, assertiveness, and communication exchanges.

I'll begin this chapter by discussing your personal responsibilities as you strive to improve your hearing capabilities, after which I'll comment on your initial experiences with hearing aids. My focus will be on how you can learn to interpret, enjoy and expand the new world of sound to which you've suddenly been exposed. I'll follow this by discussing speechreading and various exercises that can help you make the most of your residual hearing.

Finally, in the last section, I'll present some "hearing tactics," i.e., various kinds of adaptations to real-life situations aimed at improving speech comprehension. In writing this chapter, I've drawn heavily on what I've personally experienced during the many years that I've worn hearing aids (and I shudder to think what my life would be like without them).

Acknowledgment

The first and indispensable step in practicing effective communication strategies is to accept the reality of the hearing loss. Unless and until you can acknowledge its presence, openly and in a matter of fact way, you are always going to be limited in how effectively you can deal with it. A hearing loss is not something to be ashamed of; it's not a stigma that has to be hidden. *Its presence does not diminish you as a human being.* By denying or projecting your hearing difficulties onto other people's mouths ("people don't talk as clearly as they used to!"), you fool only yourself. The point is worth emphasizing. The hearing loss is there. Magical thinking, denial, not "wanting to talk about it," will not make it go away. If you don't face up to this reality, unpleasant as it may be, you're condemning yourself into a life of unnecessary stress, anxiety and isolation.

The onset of hearing loss is typically very gradual. What makes this situation particularly difficult for older people is that at first they are truly not aware that a hearing loss may be the main reason they're having communication difficulties. They can't very well deny hearing sounds that they're not aware of. This is the point where many of the conflicts between the hard of hearing person and his/her significant others first arise. It's not so much denial as disbelief; they know there are times when they can hear well. After a while, of course, the effects of the hearing loss become apparent to everyone, including the person involved. If these are ignored, then someone can truly be said to be "in denial."

Assertiveness

Once you've acknowledged the hearing loss to yourself and to others, you are then in a position to assert your communication needs in various kinds of situations. "Assertiveness" is a concept that underlies many of the specific steps I'll be suggesting later. As the person with a hearing loss, you must be willing to inform and educate others about what they have to do in order to make it easier for you to hear and understand. It may be as simple as asking the waiter in a restaurant to turn down the background music or to provide you with a written choice of the day's selections, or as involved as arranging the seats at a meeting or suggesting how your conversation partner can be a more effective communicator.

Being more assertive about your listening needs by asking others to modify their behavior does not come naturally for many people. It may mean changing the habits of a lifetime, but it can be done and it can be quite liberating (there's got to be some advantage to getting older!).

Of course, you don't have to take giant steps in the beginning. Even little ones, as long as you take enough of them, will eventually get you to your goal. You can be assertive about listening needs without being aggressive or hostile.

"Would you mind talking a little louder? I have a hearing loss and that will make it easier for me to understand you," will get better results than, "For Pete's sake, get the mud out of your mouth when you speak to me!"

When we assert our hearing needs, we're saying to somebody, "Yes, I really do want to communicate with you."

Communication Exchange

This brings up the third recurring theme in this chapter: both you and the person with whom you are talking are equally involved in a communication exchange. Presumably, this person wants to be understood as much as you want to understand. Unlike a monologue, a conversation is a two-way street. When you suggest that a seating arrangement be modified, or you inform your conversational partners what verbal modifications to make so that you can understand them, it's as much for their benefit as it is for yours. What I'm suggesting is that when you work with and help other people communicate more effectively with you, both you and others benefit. So, acknowledge your hearing loss, be *assertive about your hearing needs, and know that you are a crucial half of any communication interchange.*

Getting the Most Out of Your Hearing Aids

As a hard of hearing person you want to ensure that you're making the best use of your residual hearing. This means maximizing the benefit you're receiving through your hearing aids. Amplification is the only "therapy" that directly increases the actual amount of acoustic information available. All the training and practice procedures that are to be covered are predicated on you getting as much useful acoustic information as possible through your hearing aids. Although you should realize some immediate benefit from hearing aids, you should obtain even more help after you get used to them. Getting the most from your hearing aids requires us to consider both some general principles and some specific practice procedures.

Tenacity

Foremost—don't get discouraged! Remember that while you've had a hearing loss for a number of years and experienced the frustrations of poor hearing, for you the sounds you had been receiving seemed perfectly "normal." Now with hearing aids you're suddenly exposed to sounds that are not only louder, but a different pattern. You're going to have to reeducate your brain to accept different sound patterns as "normal." As a rather simple analogy, what you now perceive with hearing aids can be likened to someone talking English with a very different accent.

Just as it takes time for an American to get used to, for example, an Australian speaking English, or for a New Englander to comprehend the speech of someone who comes from the Deep South (and vice versa), so it will take some time for you to adjust to the amplified "accent" coming through your hearing aids.

The Adjustment Process

When you first put on your hearing aids, you're suddenly going to hear many sounds of which you previously were unaware. Many of these sounds will jog familiar memories. For others, you're going to have to consciously identify the source of the sound, either by asking someone or by honing in on it yourself. One woman in a recent hearing aid orientation group was going a little crazy with the hissing and splattering sounds she kept hearing until she realized it was coming from her frying pan. She hadn't heard the sounds of frying food for many years.

All at once you're going to be exposed to a world of sound you had forgotten, such as the whirl of the dishwasher, the whine of an electric can opener, the sounds of birds singing, or the "ting" of your microwave when the food is done. Other familiar sounds will be experienced somewhat differently and may even be disturbing, such as traffic noises in the city, the tumult in your favorite restaurant, and the screeching from your grandchildren's boombox (I'm told it's music!). It's true that it's a noisy world in which we live, and it seems to be getting noisier all the time. But it's the only world we have and it's the one in which you're going to feel more comfortable when you can more fully hear what's going on.

Expectations

Not everybody will be able to realize the same degree of benefit from hearing aids. After resisting the notion of hearing aids for years, some people, when they finally relent, expect that hearing aids will re-create their hearing abilities of fifty years ago. It doesn't work that way. While hearing aids will help most people with hearing loss, no matter how advanced a hearing aid or how skilled the hearing aid dispenser, the ultimate benefits achievable through amplification are determined by the nature of the hearing loss. Even though just about everybody with a hearing loss can obtain some benefit from hearing aids (hopefully, quite a lot), the degree of benefit will vary among individuals. Your satisfaction with hearing aids is going to depend greatly on your expectations, which should be set neither too high nor too low.

One important way to develop realistic expectations is to educate yourself about hearing loss (which is what you're doing by reading this book). Another is by talking to other people with hearing loss. A third is by working closely with the professional who fit you with hearing aids. You'll find most of them ready and willing to help you understand what you can and cannot readily achieve with hearing aids. It is important that you identify specific situations in which you appear to have the greatest difficulty, and then work with the hearing care professional to determine if there is some hearing aid

204

feature or other assistive device that can provide additional help. Such features as telephone coils, personal frequency modulation (FM) devices and television listening systems can often provide just the extra boost a person needs to overcome specific listening problems (see Appendix I). Developing realistic expectations does not mean acceptance of anything less than is possible for you.

Initial Experiences

Every hearing professional seems to have a favorite "recipe" for helping a new wearer adjust to the new world of sound produced by hearing aids. The user information booklet that comes with your hearing aids undoubtedly contains such material. I really haven't seen any wrong recipes. If you persist and work with your provider, I have no doubt that you'll eventually find your hearing aids to be helpful. Some professionals suggest that you begin by wearing hearing aids an hour or so each day, gradually increasing the time; others recommend beginning with easy listening situations (such as in quiet while talking to one person) and work yourself up to more difficult listening environments. Still others suggest just jumping right into daily use. There's nothing wrong with these recipes—they'll work if you try them diligently. But remember, it's your hearing and you can modify any rule for your convenience and comfort.

Be in Control

A key in your successful use of hearing aids is working closely with the professionals from whom you received the hearing instruments. They can't give you the full benefits of their skills unless you call upon them with your questions, comments, and experiences. For new hearing aid wearers in particular, the period right after acquiring the hearing aids is crucial. It is at this time that "Murphy's Law" (whatever can go wrong, will) seems particularly active. Most hearing aid related problems can be solved, or at least minimized, but they won't be if you don't bring them to the attention of your hearing aid practitioner. Of all the tales of woe I hear from people regarding their hearing difficulties, unsuccessful attempts to use hearing aids are surely among the most common. It really is a shame; so many people could have been greatly helped and their lives enriched if they had just persisted.

What I suggest is that you wear your hearing aids for as long each day as you feel comfortable, with the goal of wearing them all day every day. But you have to be satisfied that they're helping you hear better and they don't hurt your ears after a few hours. Sometimes, depending upon the nature of what you're hearing, you may want to remove them (e.g., at a hard rock concert, mowing the lawn on a windy day, etc.). Go ahead and take them out and don't feel guilty. Remember—you're the boss. You're in control. They're your ears!

Reeducating the Brain

What "getting used to hearing aids" really means is that you'll be undergoing a learning process. Not only will you have to get used to the hearing aids themselves, but also you will have to get used to a new pattern of sounds. For some people with long-standing hearing loss, the process of reeducating the brain can be enhanced by specific training or fitting techniques. Because you haven't heard certain sounds for a long time, the signals amplified by the hearing aids may sound strident, artificial, or just downright unpleasant. These "unnatural" or "harsh" quality sounds that you may experience can actually improve speech comprehension in the long run, but only if you can get used to them.

What the hearing aids may be doing is amplifying high frequency speech sounds (like /s/, /sh/ and /f/), elements of which you may not have heard, or have heard differently for years. Your hearing aid dispenser has a good idea of what the final amplification target should be; he or she just can't get there sometimes in one fell swoop. So, don't get discouraged if you're asked to come back for tune-ups. In fact, this may be a mark of an especially conscientious hearing care practitioner. Each time you return, your provider may perk up the high frequencies, drop the low frequencies, or do something else to help ease your adjustment to a new auditory experience. While just actively listening to people may be enough to get you used to these new sound sensations, you may also find it helpful to engage in the kinds of "listening" practice procedures that will be presented later.

Speechreading

Until recently, the preferred term for speechreading was lip-reading. We now use speechreading to emphasize the fact that when people talk, a great deal of nonverbal but important information is conveyed via facial and hand gestures, body stance, the intonation and rhythm of sentences, and the nature of the vocal emphasis placed on words and syllables. For example, the phrase "<u>Where</u> are you going?" conveys quite a different meaning than "Where are <u>you</u> going?" And "CONvict" has quite a different meaning than "conVICT," even though the two words look alike on the lips. Lip movements alone are insufficient to clarify the different meanings in these instances. What speechreading is, then, is lip-reading "plus." Our goal is not only to understand more of what a person is saying by looking at the lips, but also to be attuned to these other important sources of information. While much of this "tuning" may be unconscious, it is nevertheless very real. Speechreading will help you whether you have a mild or profound hearing loss.

If you can see a person's lips and you know the language, then you have already been speechreading—to some extent. I'll bet if I asked you if you can speechread, you'd say, "No!"

But you do!

Ask your significant other to silently mouth a month of the year (one of twelve choices). If you can't get it, try a day of the week (that is, seven rather than twelve choices). If you still don't get it (and assuming your partner's lips can be seen clearly—this is very important to check), ask this person to lip the movements for numbers "three" or "four." Nobody misses this. So, the chances are that to some extent you have already been speechreading as long as you can observe the lips of the speaker. But you should do even better if you know the general principles of speechreading.

Speechreading Principles

Visibility

The first general principle is that you must be able to see the lips of the person talking. Now this not only sounds simplistic, but positively insulting! Of course one has to see the lips in order to speechread. But you would be surprised how many people with hearing loss who need and can benefit from speechreading do not observe the lips of their conversational partners. They may look them "right in the eye" or simply stare off to one side.

The lip movements we're trying to pick up are minuscule, rapid, and very fleeting. Since our vision is most acute at the point of focus, our best chance of perceiving these cues is by looking right at the lips. For example, our peripheral vision should be sufficient to detect facial expressions, hand gestures, body stance, and so forth because they are larger movements. Try it. Look at someone's lips and note that you can also see the expression on his or her face as well as any hand movements.

Think about the implications of these simple rules. You will not be able to speechread when:

- in the dark
- a person's back is turned
- you're far from a person
- your visual acuity is poor (so, pay as much attention to your vision as to your hearing)
- a person's mouth is covered
- your conversational partner wears a full mustache and beard
- light is in your eyes
- the head of the person you're talking to is shadowed

In other words, any situation that reduces the visibility of the lips is going to interfere with speechreading. How often have you, or people you know, made an extra effort, perhaps unconsciously, to ensure that you can see the person who's talking? If you have, you've been speechreading, even though you may not have known it.

Restricting Lip Movements

Anything that interferes with the movements of the lips is also going to interfere with speechreading. Some people seem unable to talk unless they have a pencil or the frame of eyeglasses jutting out of their mouth. Other people talk as if they were practicing to be ventriloquists—their lips hardly move at all. And some people seem to talk with a perpetual smile, making speechreading almost impossible because of the way the smile distorts lip movements. In a few of these instances, a little assertiveness may help, such as "Please take the pencil out of your mouth."

But for others it's a losing battle. (Although I've often been tempted, I have not yet said "Wipe that smile off your face!" to someone with a perennial grin.) Because of the wide variations in the size and movement of the lips while talking, there will be large individual variations in the speechreadability of someone's lips. For people with whom you have a continuing relationship, it's worth reminding them to use more lip movements while talking. Sometimes this works quite well. For the tight-lipped stranger, this may be a futile endeavor. It may be easier to change the world than the way some people talk. So, be realistic. You can't win them all.

Familiarity with the Language

You can't speechread unless you know the language. This also sounds quite simplistic, and in a way it is. If you're trying to speechread someone talking in a foreign language, of course you won't be able to. But what this brings up is the notion of predictability. Since only about 30 percent of the sounds in the English language are clearly visible on the lips, even in the best of circumstances there are lots of gaps that have to be filled in. This is not quite as imposing a task as it may appear, as long as you and the person you're talking to share a common language. English is very redundant, with many linguistic and situational cues that can help you correctly predict some words you otherwise couldn't. For example, try filling in the blanks in the following sentences:

A. Please put the dish on the _____.
B. He hit a home _____ in the last _____.
C. Where are you _____?
D. It snowed again last _____.
E. I just heard the weather report. They are _____ a major _____ tonight.

In sentence "A," someone could be saying "floor" or "bookcase," rather than "table," but this is unlikely. Sentence "E" is an example of how a previous sentence (or sentences) can improve predictability. The words are "predicting" and "storm." Now—wasn't that easy?

Native language speakers do this kind of thing unconsciously. No matter what language you've grown up with, you can (or could prior to the onset of your hearing loss) effortlessly understand verbal messages. Don't you often fill in the last part of people's conversations before they finish? This is the kind of predictability I mean. If you're not listening to your native language, then you will have more difficulty making these predictions (as well as more difficulty understanding speech in noise or other difficult listening situations).

Topic Restrictions

The ability to speechread improves when you can reduce the conversational possibilities. When you go to the bank, a travel agency, a municipal office, shop in a clothing store, or talk to a co-worker regarding a particular project, the topics are likely to be limited by the context. I don't suppose you talk about certificates of deposit in the clothing store, or the weather in Italy at the bank. Basically, "topic restrictions" are another way of employing linguistic predictability.

This is not something you necessarily do consciously. However, the fact that topic restrictions do enter into almost any conversation should make it easier for you to speechread and to keep from making bad guesses. If it makes no sense at all, it probably wasn't the message! Yes, a lot of guessing does take place, and sometimes, as has happened to me, I guess wrong (with occasional embarrassment but just as often, a laugh for everybody). Still, I would rather guess and keep the conversation going than give up.

It's the Message Not the Medium

When you're engaged in a conversation, don't focus on speechreading particular sounds or words. Instead, attend to the message—the meaning of what the other person is trying to convey. If you consciously try to analyze the minuscule, rapid, and fleeting movements of the lips, you're going to be three sentences behind before you figure out the missing sounds or words—if you ever do. Many books on speechreading spend an inordinate amount of time describing how the different sounds of speech are made. Speechreading successfully, however, does not require you to identify all the sounds a person forms on his or her lips. What it means is that you're able to comprehend what the person is saying.

Listen to the message rather than focusing on how the different sounds appear on the lips. Because so many of the sounds of speech are either invisible or are formed exactly the same way as other sounds, even the most skilled speechreader cannot identify all of them. What they do, and what you must do, is use your knowledge of the language and your awareness of topic restrictions to fill in the gaps. By focusing on the message rather than specific movements, you'll find that subsequent sentences may clarify words that you may have missed.

Hearing

One crucial principle in speechreading is the necessity for you to use your residual hearing as well as you can. Now, this seems like a contradiction! If we're talking about speechreading, why bring up hearing? Well, how often are you talking to someone while you're not wearing your hearing aids? Maybe late at night or early in the morning, but at most other times you're likely to be wearing them. And why would you not wear them if you know they help you? Normally, then, when conversing with other people, you're going to depend on both speechreading and hearing. And that's fine. Because your goal is to understand speech as well as you can, you should use whatever cues are available to help you realize this goal.

As I mentioned earlier, many of the sounds in English are completely invisible on the lips. For example, look in the mirror while saying the word "key." It can be said with no movement at all. This is the kind of word that requires context in order to understand.

For example, to the teenager in the house, "No you can't have the _____ to the car!" Context is the only way the word can be understood. Now, while you're still in front of the mirror, silently say the words /pan/, /ban/, and /man/. They all look alike, don't they? This is where hearing comes in. Fortunately, it's relatively easy to hear the difference between the /b/, /p/, and /m/ sounds, since /b/ is voiced, /p/ is voiceless and /m/ is a nasal sound (also voiced).

In other words, much of what you can't see, you can hear. This is an important principle. It turns out that there are many speech sounds that are very difficult to tell apart visually, and yet are relatively easy to distinguish through hearing (i.e., while the /t/, /d/, and /n/ sounds look identical, they can be differentiated through hearing). Conversely, other sounds that are difficult to hear (like /s/, /f/, /t/, and /th/) are relatively easy to speechread. So, what we find is that vision and audition provide complementary information. What is lacking or difficult to perceive in one modality can often be picked up in the other. Therefore, depending only on speechreading, or only on hearing, limits your ability to communicate.

In real-life situations, there are always going to be variations in how well you can see and hear someone talking. Noise will tend to mask out many speech sounds and reduce the amount of information you get through hearing. This forces you to depend more on visual cues in order to understand a spoken message. But because the loudness and type of noise constantly vary, these changes will cause your ability to understand speech to vary as well. In some situations you may have to rely almost entirely on vision to understand speech, while in other situations, you may be able to understand even without looking at the speaker.

Therefore, you have to be prepared for an unpredictable

amount of hearing information due to varying noise backgrounds, as well as unpredictable visual cues. By using both vision and audition as much as possible, and any other sources of information, *most* hard of hearing people can comprehend *most* of what *most* people say in *most* situations. I'm qualifying because there will inevitably be times when you miss part or almost all of a conversation. This will happen. What I'm suggesting is that you think positively. Think of the occasions you can understand rather than the times you can't. That is, the glass is half full, not half empty!

Practice Procedures

There have been hundreds of books and articles purporting to teach people how to speechread, often extolling some specific theory and providing lots of practice material. Personally, I find the practice material more helpful than the theories. Practice will help improve just about any skill. I personally had experienced the benefits of speechreading practice several years ago. For about a month I could not use my hearing aids because of an infection in both ear canals. All I could depend upon was speechreading (with an 85-95 dB loss in both ears, without hearing aids I'm functionally deaf).

Ordinarily, I'm a very poor speechreader. After several weeks of trying to communicate without hearing, mainly with my wife, I found my ability to speechread her noticeably improving. I still couldn't carry on an extended conversation by speechreading alone, but at least in context I was able to carry on abbreviated conversations. (We did cheat once in a while and use finger spelling to clarify difficult words!)

So, it's very possible that speechreading practice, with and without sound, wherever and with whomever you do it, is going to help you improve your understanding of spoken messages. In addition to the informal practice you get every day when you talk to people (and don't underestimate the value of these experiences!) formal training activities can also help. One creative such exercise, termed tracking procedures, is practiced "live," with a communication partner. Don't be discouraged by the professional jargon. These are basically exercises that require you to comprehend segments of speech before proceeding to subsequent segments. In other words, you're required to "track" through a conversation in a sequential manner. The tracking exercises can be structured so that they incorporate speechreading, auditory training, as well as communication repair strategies. Let me explain how this works.

You are sitting across from your conversational partner. The room is well lit and you're relaxed. (It's going to be fun!) This person has selected a paragraph as practice material; it can be from the newspaper, from a magazine article or book, or specific material related to one's vocation or interests. Whatever material is selected, it's important that the sentences follow each other in some kind of logical sequence. You should be informed of the general content or topic of the paragraph, as would be the case in real life.

Now, while using a soft voice and normal, not exaggerated lip movements (adding noise via television or radio will enhance the realism of the exercise), your partner should read the first sentence of the paragraph to you. Did you get it all? Did you get any of it? Your job is to repeat whatever you understood of the sentence, guessing when you're not sure. You probably made some errors but also got some words correct.

If you missed any part of the sentence, the first step is for your partner to repeat the whole sentence again, verbatim. You may or may not get it all this time. If not, what your partner has to do is emphasize the parts you missed, increasing the duration, exaggerating the pronunciation, and so forth.

For example, "Did you remember to shut off the WATER when you left the house?"

Your partner keeps doing this until you get the entire sentence correct. At the beginning of the paragraph, to get the process going, you may need a few more cues. If you repeatedly miss a part of the sentence, despite the extra emphasis, your partner should give you extra hints.

For example, "The word begins with an /s/ sound," or "It's the name of a country in Europe." Paraphrasing the sentence before going back to the original version also can help. In this exercise (unlike a later one), it is the partner who has to determine the correct "communication repair" strategies.

The point is for you to be able to repeat the sentence correctly, using whatever clues the partner provides, including raised voice or writing the words down as last resorts. Then your partner should repeat the sentence, even though you now know it, but this time followed by the second sentence—the one you don't yet know. The more sentences you comprehend in a paragraph, the more the internal linguistic cues will help you understand subsequent sentences. The more practice you get, the quicker you'll be going through the process. This is a wonderful exercise for teaching concentration and identifying specific sounds and words that give you the most difficulty.

Practicing "Communication Repair" Strategies

In this exercise, you take the responsibility for "repairing" the broken communication during the tracking exercise. What has broken down, of course, is the communication exchange. You didn't quite get the entire intended message. When you don't understand, the person you're talking to doesn't really know why or what he or she can do to correct the situation. But you should know what aspect of a person's speech made it difficult for you to understand, and you can advise your conversational partner how to communicate more effectively with you. The rationale is simple. In real life conversation, asking "what?" or "huh?" when you don't understand doesn't often help very much. Mostly what people will do when they hear these expressions is to simply say the whole thing over and over again, maybe just as softly, quickly, or poorly articulated.

In this exercise, your task is to try to figure out why you missed what you did, and then to ask your partner to make specific modifications in his or her speech. Maybe you don't need the entire sentence repeated; maybe all you didn't get was the last word. So you ask the person to repeat only the portion you missed. Or maybe your partner looked down while talking, slurred a particular word, or talked too fast. With a creative collaborator, you can simulate many real-life situations. Your goal is to practice "communication repair" strategies enough so that you can utilize them in everyday life. Like asking a ticket agent at an airport to look at you when talking, or to talk a little louder, slower, and so forth. When you help the person you're talking with to be a more effective communicator with you, you're applying the three themes I spoke about earlier: you're acknowledging your hearing loss, being assertive about your communication needs, and placing equal responsibility for the communication exchange on the person with whom you're talking.

Listening Practice (Auditory Training)

If we've learned anything in audiology in the past 50 years, it's that the hard of hearing person's perception of speech is not immutable. This has been dramatically illustrated to us in recent years by deaf people who have received cochlear implants (see Chapter 8 Q&A #8). People initially report some strange auditory sensations that they're unable to identify or use. After a while, however, learning takes place. The brain "links up" to the acoustic environment and strange sounds become identifiable. While new users of hearing aids may not experience anything quite so dramatic, improvements in speech perception do take place, sometimes quite rapidly and sometimes slowly. Focused listening practice can help accelerate this process as well as stimulate the maximum use of a person's residual hearing.

With a Partner

Adaptations of the previously described tracking procedure can serve as helpful "auditory training" procedures. In the auditory version, your partner reads the material for you to repeat while his or her lips are covered (no visual cues). For most people, this is still going to be too easy.

Think about situations in which you have the most difficulty understanding the spoken word—in noise, right? Okay, then that's how you should structure the tracking procedures. Perhaps the best kind of "noise" to use is narration on audiocassettes, such as books on tape. This will make the listening task difficult, as it should be. Use these recordings as background sounds and not as training stimuli. In a later section, you'll see how the same recordings can be used for self-administered auditory training.

The first sentence is read. If you miss part or all of it, your partner should, in this order:

- repeat it verbatim;
- repeat it stressing the words you missed;
- if you still miss it, the sentence should be rephrased, but then go back to the original version for you to repeat;
- and finally, let you see and hear the sentence if you still missed it.

After you get the first sentence, your partner should then read the second one and continue the process throughout the entire paragraph. How long should you do this? I suggest no more than 15-30 minutes in the beginning (as long as you and your partner feel comfortable). As you well know, trying to listen under adverse circumstances can be very fatiguing.

Self-Administered Auditory Training

Getting and keeping a cooperative partner can be quite a challenge. After a while, you may run out of cooperative partners! Remember, though, the purpose of the training procedure is not to endanger relationships, but to foster good listening habits! You can advance toward the same goal working by yourself, using available audiocassette materials that come with written scripts.

Years ago I used this technique to help convince severely hearing-impaired children and their parents and teachers that the children could use and benefit from their residual hearing. While we recorded our own material and wrote our own scripts, this is no longer necessary. There's a lot of this kind of material now—for example, books on tape, and audio tapes developed for second language learners that include a word-for-word written transcript. Check with your local bookstore or reference librarian. You'll find that there are recorded poems, short stories, formal lectures, and so on that include verbatim written transcripts. You could apply this technique, or a variation on this theme, in a few ways:

1) Most easily, all you do is listen to the tape while following the written script. This will get you used to hearing aid amplified sounds, and you may even enjoy the recording! But this doesn't present you with much of an auditory challenge.

2) A more difficult procedure would be to listen to a short paragraph and then read the script. What did you miss just by listening? Even though you may have missed some words, did the meaning come through? With some English as a Second Language (ESL) tapes, you're required to answer written questions to determine if you got the basic point. In addition to answering these questions, you can also check to see if you could comprehend all the words. Try to analyze the words you consistently missed—did they incorporate specific sound elements (like some high frequency consonants) of which you should be aware?

3) An even more challenging method is to make two copies of the same script, one for the exercise and one for verification. Ask someone else to randomly whiteout several words in each sentence in one of the copies, starting with just one word in the first sentence, then increasing the number of words eliminated in later sentences. Some of the words should be predictable from the context; others, like proper nouns, much less so. Stress the fact that you want both "easy to hear" and "hard to hear" words removed with whiteout. Your

task is to listen to this edited script and fill in the omitted words. After you listen to the entire page, you then check the original copy to determine how well you did. This process will help you "reeducate" your hearing (and brain) as you become a more focused listener.

Carry-over

All training procedures are designed to prepare you to use these techniques in real life, outside of the practice sessions. If your training partner is someone you talk with all the time, these training activities can eventually carry over to your real-life verbal interchanges. There's some good research to indicate that extra effort on the part of the person talking does improve speech comprehension for hard of hearing people. It's called "clear speech" or what Grandma has been telling the kids to do for centuries (slow down a bit, pronounce words more clearly, speak just a little louder).

But even strangers and infrequent communication partners want you to understand what they are saying. You can be assertive in such situations without being aggressive. Put the burden on yourself. Say, for example, "Could you talk a little slower please. I have a hearing loss and it would make it easier for me to understand you."

You must acknowledge your hearing loss in order to employ these communication strategies effectively. Don't bluff and pretend you understand. You no doubt already know you can damage a relationship, misunderstand important instructions, and get into a heap of trouble. When it comes to important instructions, dates, names, and so forth, even if you think you understand, make sure you clarify just to be certain, by repeating what you think you heard. "Did you say two blue pills every three hours and three white pills every two hours?" It can make a difference!

Hearing Tactics

"Hearing tactics" is a term used to describe environmental manipulations that make it easier for you to understand other people. I don't mean being sneaky or manipulative in the usual sense of the word. You're reading this book because you're having difficulty in many situations and you want to do something about it. While the procedures described earlier will help, they are not the only steps you can take to help yourself. Most likely, as you interact with other people in a number of situations, you're still going to have some difficulty hearing everything that's going on.

Using hearing tactics like military tactics means you plan ahead, marshal your resources, and engage the "enemy"—the difficult communication situation. Now, no hearing tactic, or any hearing device for that matter, will eliminate all of your hearing problems. But you can take a giant step toward reducing many of them by understanding how you can exert more control over the communicative situation. Several examples follow.

Move closer

Always try to move closer to the person talking (but do respect their "personal space!") This is an underestimated but valuable technique. For example, in the average room, if you're eight feet from someone speaking and you can move to within four feet of this person, you've increased the sound pressure at the microphone of your hearing aids by 6 dB. If you can get within two feet of the speaker, then the increase is 12 dB — a rather significant boost. I really don't recommend getting much closer unless you have a "special relationship" with this individual!

While it's true that some modern hearing aids will compensate for distance by providing more amplification of weaker sounds, and less for the stronger sounds, they will also amplify strong and weak background noises in a similar fashion. Better comprehension results when the sound you want to hear is located close to the hearing aid microphone, whether this sound is a person talking, a television set, radio, or anything else. This will improve the speech to noise ratio (the intensity level of the speech relative to the noise) which is perhaps the most important factor underlying your speech perception.

Quiet the Room

This is a principle that applies just about every place you go. When you walk into a restaurant for a relaxing meal and find that the young staff is playing loud music through the PA system, what do you do? Here's where assertiveness pays off. Many young people seem completely unaware that there is loud music in the background—this all seems very normal to them.

When it's explained that the music makes speech comprehension virtually impossible for the person with a hearing loss, more often than not they graciously comply with the request to lower the volume. Hopefully, after a few such requests, they may learn to appreciate the "sounds of silence." Wouldn't it be nice to have "noise-free" areas in the same way we now have "smoke-free" restaurants?

When you arrive, look or ask for the quietest table. The hostess usually knows. Don't sit in the middle of a room with parties all around you, although you can seat yourself in the center of your group where it's easy for you to see and hear everyone. Stay away from any extra noise-producing areas such as the kitchen, background piano music, an air conditioner or heating system. Better yet, look for places to eat that encourage private conversations; restaurants do differ in their sensitivity to noise.

Many people feel that they have to have the stereo turned on when entertaining people in their home. A gentle reminder to turn it down or even off usually suffices. In a family gathering, the youngsters may have the television set turned up while ignoring it; if it's your house, pull the plug and/or move the youngsters to another room. If it's not your house, try diplomacy or try to move your personal conversation to a quieter area in the house. Whatever house you happen to be in, make sure you have a good sight-line to all the guests. Don't sit at the end of a long couch. You won't be able to see or hear the person at the other end. If only a small group is involved, try to get some conversational "rules" established. If these people are friends, you can ask that only one person talk at a time. "Cross-conversation" presents one of the most difficult situations for people with hearing loss.

Senior centers and retirement homes, particularly those that serve meals, often present a challenging communication environment. In such places, the acoustical conditions can be improved by:

- acoustical treatment on ceilings and walls
- rugs, if possible, on the floor
- or rubber coasters on chair and table legs
- soft material, such as felt, on dining tables under the tablecloths to reduce the clattering sounds of dishes and silverware
- sitting at a smaller (4-person) rather than larger (8-person) table during meals and other activities

Advance Planning

Do some anticipatory planning for any activity. For example, before you attend any large-area listening situation (theater, lecture, house of worship, etc.) call ahead to see if an assistive listening device is available. These devices basically transmit the sound from its source to special receivers (FM radio, infra-red, or the telephone coil in your hearing aid). They enhance acoustical clarity of sounds that emanate from loudspeakers some distance from you.

Most such places are required to have such listening devices available, according to the Americans with Disabilities Act (ADA). Houses of worship are an exception, yet many provide such devices as a moral obligation. I personally would not attend any large area listening event without ensuring that such devices were available. Without one, I either don't know what's going on or I'm straining so hard to hear that I don't enjoy the activity or performance.

Microphone Technique

Even if assistive listening devices are available in an auditorium, listening problems can still occur, particularly if the sound source comes from someone using a microphone. What I have observed over the years is an abysmal ignorance of proper microphone technique, even by people who should know better.

In any large area listening situation, the lack of good microphone technique is often the weakest link in the communication chain. What seems to happen is that talkers get so wrapped up in what they're saying, they forget that there's a microphone on the podium. Most of these are low-sensitivity microphones, requiring a talker to be within four to six inches of it for effective pick-up. Sometimes if it's a hand-held microphone, many people wave it around as if it were a baton or a pointer—everywhere but close to their mouth. So what do you do?

- You arrive a little earlier and remind the event organizer, the speaker or the minister, of the necessity for the speaker to stay close to the microphone while talking.
- During the talk, some speakers are going to walk away from the microphone still speaking. You ask loudly (but politely) for the speaker to move closer to the microphone. Other people in the audience will appreciate your assertiveness because of their own hearing difficulty.
- If a lapel instead of a podium microphone is available, ask that it be used and pinned close to the person's mouth.
- If there's a public question and answer period after the talk and you can't hear the questions, don't suffer in silence. Ask for the questions to be repeated before answers are given. Remember that you're probably not the only one in the audience who can't hear the questions.

In a recent hearing aid orientation group, I heard of an excellent example of how a bit of assertiveness can help many other people in the audience. One of the participants complained that he never heard the homilies prepared by the same two women in his church. Their voices were soft and they typically sat two feet or so away from the microphone. Every Sunday, he said he just sat there and waited for them to finish, not understanding a word.

His normal hearing wife then piped up and said, "I never understand them either and I don't think anyone else can!"

Before the next service, the husband asked the two women to talk right into the microphone as he was having difficulty understanding them. That Sunday, not only my client, but everyone heard the women loud and clear.

Wrap up

In this church anecdote, we have an example of the three themes with which I began this chapter. The hard of hearing person had to *acknowledge* his hearing loss, had to *be assertive* in approaching speakers, and the *effort served the purposes of both parties* in the communication exchange. The lesson in this example is that you, as a hard of hearing person, must be more than a passive recipient of hearing "services." You have to take more control over your own listening needs. Work closely with your hearing healthcare professionals. They have information and skills that will help you.

No—magic wands are not available to "wave" away your hearing loss, but with the appropriate use of modern technology and the judicious use of appropriate communication strategies, you can go a long way in reducing the impact hearing loss is having in your life.

APPENDIX I
Assistive Listening Devices [ALDs]

Assistive Listening Devices (ALDs) describe equipment that amplifies sound and enhances your ability to hear. As a result, your hearing world becomes a more pleasant experience through less strain and frustration. If you have a hearing loss of even a mild degree, you can benefit substantially from many of these devices.

Many ALDs operate in conjunction with your hearing aids through a built-in telecoil switch, commonly identified on BTE hearing aids with a "T." On In-The-Ear models you may simply find a toggle switch that triggers the telecoil function. This allows activation of a small, harmless, electromagnetic field through which the external assistive listening device can operate with your hearing aid. While some hearing aids now have electromagnetic connections built into the circuit without you having to do anything, this is certainly the future trend in all such technology.

Most BTE hearing aids can accommodate what is called a Direct Audio Input (DAI). This system comes with a special manufacturer-designed boot (a coupler) that clips around your aid enabling you to plug into and listen to TV, radio, stereo, DVD, FM or conference system. In-The-Ear hearing aids can also utilize direct audio input if they have the optional "T" switch on them. The DAI is a wonderful advantage to you because it offers the cleanest, clearest sound reception. However, it does require that you have a "T" position on your hearing aid by means of which your target listening system is linked to your aid through an electromagnetic field. Ask your hearing care provider about how this option may work for you.

Some ALDs do not require that you even wear hearing aids in order to benefit from amplified sound such as television and some telephone amplifiers. You will find a wide variety of devices in this section that represent only a small sampling of what is actually available—from telephone and alerting products to television and signaling devices. These products will enhance your hearing ability, resulting in less stress, increased clarity and audibility.

Many of these devices can actually solve hearing problems. Something as simple as not blasting the television (by having your own remote amplifier) has solved many an argument and household disruption.

Your initial thought might be, "Why would I need these since I just purchased a top-of-the-line set of hearing aids!"

The answer is that hearing aids are designed to amplify human speech. You may derive some added benefits from them, such as hearing the car radio better, or the ticking of a clock, but they may not adequately amplify specific auditory needs such as television, or the doorbell or telephone ringing from another room. There are many alternative amplified systems designed that will nicely augment your hearing aids, allowing you to hear sounds other than speech.

To better understand the development of ALDS, it might be helpful to have some background. In the 1970s, most telephone amplification equipment was issued at no charge to accounts under American Telephone and Telegraph companies. However, since "Ma-Bel's" break-up, a tremendous flood of market possibilities opened up for new companies and products. This was a great boon to all who had hearing loss, as the rather fierce competition for this narrow market kept the prices of these products affordable.

Something you need to realize is that not all hearing care practitioners carry ALDs in their offices. This is largely due to the very narrow profit margins manufacturers and distributors allow. In a busy office, many practitioners may feel ALDs are a distraction to their primary clinical functions. Don't be dismayed. Ask your hearing care practitioner for names of companies you can directly contact. Many practitioners have giveaway catalogs in their office. You can also go on the Internet and search for *assistive listening devices*, locating company catalogs online and ordering.

Because wireless communication (such as cell phones) has come into being as a viable and important avenue of communication, this appendix will include some cell phone items that will enhance your ability to hear.

However, it's worth mentioning here that cell phone designs have not really kept up with the personal needs of people with hearing loss. Typically, you could find cell phones are not loud enough and there's too much interference with background noises. As of this writing in 2004, the FCC is moving slowly to mandate laws for hearing aid compatibility with cell phones. This means they are making strong suggestions for manufacturers to operate by in order to establish better compliance between digital cell phones and hearing aids.

In the final analysis, it may be up to you to discover what augmentative products will best serve your cell phone needs. You might find that your most optimal hearing is derived from "hands free" speaker-phone style cell phones whereby you have the advantage of hearing with both ears along with your hearing aids.

Something to keep in mind is there are a number of companies that manufacture or distribute very similar devices, particularly in the area of alarm clocks, television amplified equipment, and telephone ringer-amplified and receiver-amplified products. For example, for standard telephone receiver handsets, several items are available to clip over the earpiece of the receiver to allow you significant audio boost on incoming calls. Such "portability" offers you the convenience of carrying this in your pocket wherever you go and using it on any telephone when you travel (worldwide). Others are fixed units built into the receiver handset and are sold as a single device that replaces your current receiver. And still other products are manufactured that connect into your telephone line (wire) and provide amplification this way.

Naturally, there are a variety of prices, depending on which products you select from a particular company. With respect to prices, none are listed in this section because they change from year to year. Most products in this section are under $100; some are up to $300; and the more sophisticated amplified systems can run as high as $1000 or more.

The names of companies cited as having provided a photo courtesy of their organization is done to allow hearing healthcare professionals who might not be familiar with these devices and companies to have an opportunity to contact them and establish an in-house corner of their office to display some of them. You can also find ALD distributors on the Internet.

Finally, something of importance you should know is the warranty coverage you have on particular products. For example, some items carry only a one-year warranty while others have five years. Some companies have no fees for returns while others may charge you a "restocking fee." Make these inquiries *before you make the purchase.*

Good luck!

DISCLAIMER: Listing of products should in no way be construed as an endorsement of any company, product or device by the Publisher, the Editor or any contributing authors of this book. Any purchases of these devices are a responsibility between you and the company from which you make the purchase. Also, bear in mind that these products were not rated in any way. That is, it cannot be assumed that a particular product listed here is any better or worse than a comparable item available elsewhere.

Alerting Devices

Bed Shaker
is a device that can be connected to an alarm clock to awaken you by fitting under and vibrating your bed or pillow. It is an excellent system for especially heavy sleepers, and gives you the most assurance of waking up on time.

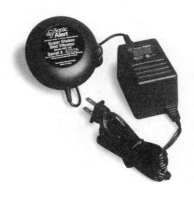

[Photo Courtesy of General Technologies]

Vibrating Wristwatch

is a multi-purpose watch that can be preset to a specific time to vibrate and remind you to take your medication, attend a meeting, make a phone call, and so forth. It comes with an audio alarm setting as well. Additional features include a

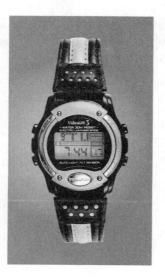

99-hour stop watch function, 99-hour countdown timer with count repeat mode, and LCD displays day of week and month. It uses a long life lithium battery, and comes with a one-year warranty.

[Photo Courtesy of LS&S, LLC]

Sonic Alert Wireless Doorbell/Telephone Signaler

plugs into any modular telephone jack and does not draw any phone line power that could prevent some phones from ringing. It has a selectable number of flashes to alert you, works at home with all intercom systems, flash codes can be set at different rates to identify back door, front door, etc., and has built-in chimes for hearing members of the family.

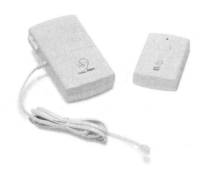

[Photo Courtesy of Sound Clarity, Inc.]

Gentex 710-CSW Smoke Detector

is a photoelectric single station smoke detector designed to give reliable early warning of the presence of smoke where both audible and visual alarms are required. (This model is hard-wired so you would need an electrician to hook it up.) Standard features include 177 candela rating (very bright strobe light); solid state 90 dB horn (very loud); full function test switch (easy for you to test that it is working); flashes 60 times per minute; quick-disconnect wiring harness; mounting hardware for wall; tandem connection up to 6 detectors per system; AC-powered also available; one year warranty.

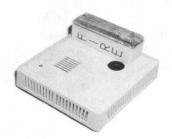

[Photo Courtesy of Harris Communications, Inc.]

Sonic Boom Alarm Clock

is a unique clock that can wake up even heavy sleepers. When the alarm goes off, you can select to wake up to any combination of loud pulsating audio alarm, flashing lights, or shaking bed (vibrator sold separately). The vibrator can produce steady or pulsating vibration pattern for maximum effectiveness. There is a test button on the unit to explore which combination of flashing lights, shaking bed or loud pulsating audio alarm will work best for you.

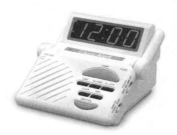

[Photo Courtesy of Sound Clarity, Inc.]

Enhanced Listening Systems

Sound Wizard II

is a complete communication system. It utilizes either a directional microphone (for one-to-one conversation in noise) or omni-directional microphones (for groups). Dual headset jacks allow two people simultaneous use with good clarity in noise. The powerful amplifier and tone control allows you to hear better in many situations. It can be connected to your existing telephone and is compatible with headsets, earbuds, neckloops, silhouettes, and external speakers for use in movie theaters and public facilities. Two AA batteries included (for 200 hours of life), with a five-year warranty.

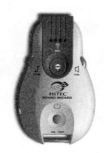

[Photo Courtesy of Hitec Group International, Inc.]

PocketTalker Pro

is an easy-to-use, portable, battery-operated amplifier that can improve your ability to communicate in difficult listening situations. It utilizes a sensitive directional microphone that can be placed close to the sound source to minimize background noise. It comes with 2 AA batteries that provide up to 100 hours of use. Included in the package is a microphone extension cord for TV listening with optional links for use with hearing aids, telephones and neckloops. It comes with a five-year warranty.

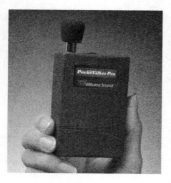

[Photo Courtesy of Adco Hearing Products, Inc.]

Room Amplification System

amplifies a person's voice in a room with other hard-of-hearing people if you need more power than your hearing aids provide. It distributes sounds equally throughout the room by means of 4 speakers with hanging brackets that can be used in different speaker arrays. A wireless microphone allows for ease of movement throughout the room for the primary person speaking (such as a teacher), and the two-channel amplifier makes team teaching easy. Among a number of items, the system includes a rechargeable battery; an amplifier; wireless transmitter and receiver; and one neckloop.

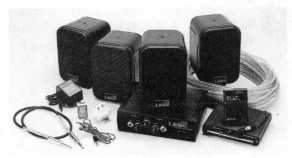

[Photo Courtesy of Harris Communications, Inc.]

FM, Infrared and Loop Systems

Nady 351 VR Personal (Wireless) FM System

gives you clear, professional sounding high fidelity audio without distracting ambient noise from the environment and is made for commercial video sound recording. The operating range is up to 200' even in the most adverse conditions, and up to 500' line-of-sight. It is available in 5 different frequencies and can be effectively used in multiple system set-ups.

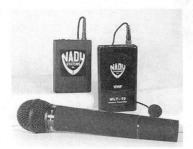

[Photo Courtesy of General Technologies]

Personal FM System "Hearing Helper"

broadcasts the speaker's voice directly to the ears of individual listeners. While the person speaking wears a compact transmitter and microphone, listeners use portable receivers and earphones to hear the presentation clearly and easily,

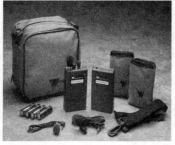

[Photo Courtesy of Adco Hearing Products, Inc.]

even from the back of the room. It helps listeners overcome background noise, reverberation, and distance from the speaker in classrooms and small groups, thus maximizing their ability to hear and understand. It operates on 2 AA batteries and includes a transmitter and portable receiver.

Personal FM (PPA 375) Public Address System

features the new T35 high performance transmitter; powerful microprocessor; sleek digital display; and easy-to-use menu controls. The T35 configures itself to the appropriate setting, taking the guesswork out of complicated audio installation. Operating up to 1000 feet, the T35 is ideal for auditoriums,

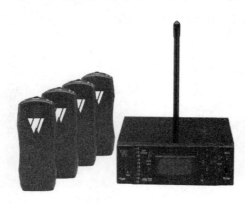

theaters, or other large venues where excellent coverage area is essential. The system includes 4 impact-resistant R35 single-channel receivers. The R35 receiver will operate up to 80 hours for long-lasting performance!

[Photo Courtesy of Adco Hearing Products, Inc.]

ICON-TR60 Infrared Conference Emitter
is an advanced, wireless, self-contained infrared emitter combining portability with ease of use. Great for conference and boardroom meetings, group therapy, jury deliberation rooms, or situations around tables where it's difficult to hear.

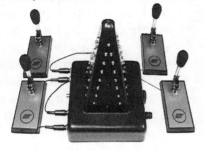

When multiple microphones are used, the one nearest the person speaking sets the level of volume for the others, which has the effect of reducing background noise whenever anyone speaks into any microphones.

[Photo Courtesy of Harris Communications, Inc.]

Telephone Devices

The Teletalker
is designed to improve speech understanding over the telephone. It combines a powerful amplifier with a sophisticated signal processing circuit to enhance phone signal quality. To enhance or amplify a call, press the amplify button, then adjust the volume and enhancement controls for maximum comfort and clarity. When you hang up, it automatically returns to normal operation, protecting others from unintended amplification. The phone lets you boost high

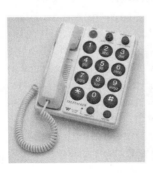

[Photo Courtesy of Adco Hearing Products, Inc.]

frequencies as needed to emphasize speech sounds that contribute to maximum understanding. The anti-feedback circuit permits full use of amplification without problems of howling, feedback or distortion. It can be used with a telecoil–equipped hearing aid coupled with the handset speaker, and comes with a five–year warranty.

Walker Clarity High Frequency Telephone Amplifier

is designed to help people with high frequency hearing loss hear words clearer, not just louder. It amplifies incoming calls up to 25+ dB when the boost button is activated. Also, it is compatible with standard and electronic phones, single or multi-lines, and has a low battery indicator. It cannot be used with dial-in handset receivers. It requires 2 AAA batteries (not included) and comes with a one-year warranty.

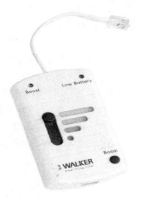

[Photo Courtesy of
LS&S, LLC]

V-Tech 2400-A Cordless Amplified Phone

utilizes 2.4 GHz digital transmission, providing outstanding operating range while maintaining clarity for people with hearing loss who need help in noisy situations. Incoming voices are amplified up to 30 dB. The phone is hearing aid compatible with a powerful t-coil built into the handset. The phone also has a 3.5mm amplified stereo jack for an optional neckloop and a 2.5mm non-amplified jack for an optional telephone headset. It has 50 number caller ID; call waiting; multi-level volume control; time/date; hands-free belt clip; low battery and out-of-range indicators; and a one-year warranty.

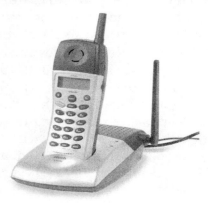

[Photo Courtesy of Hitec
Group International, Inc.]

HA-40 In-Line Telephone Amplifier

is a powerful in-line amplifier with a tone selector, allowing words to be heard loud and clear. A separate boost feature blocks out background noise and feedback for maximum amplification. To achieve the full 40 dB of amplification, you must hold down the "BOOST" button while listening and then release the button when talking. Without the "BOOST" feature

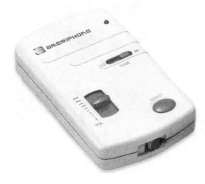

activated, the unit operates as a powerful 30 dB amplifier with the additional 10 dB of assistance available only when needed. It will not work on phones where the dial pad is in the handset, or on cordless phones. This item includes batteries, and comes with a manufacturer's one-year warranty.

[Photo Courtesy of Hitec Group International, Inc.]

PA 25 Portable Telephone Amplifier

increases volume of incoming voices up to 25 dB, easily straps to most any telephone handset style, ideal to use with payphones, cordless or cellular telephones, lightweight and extremely portable, and hearing aid compatible. It comes with 2 AAA batteries, a carrying case, and a six-month manufacturer's warranty.

[Photo Courtesy of Sound Clarity, Inc.]

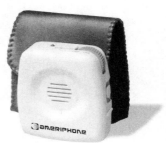

Walker Clarity Extra Loud Telephone Ringer

allows you to hear the telephone ring up to 95 dB. A red light indicator also alerts you to incoming calls. It comes with a built-in surge protector, requires no batteries or AC hook-up, is compatible with all analog phone systems, and requires no special jacks. It carries a one-year warranty.

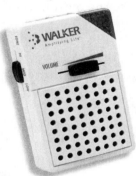

[Photo Courtesy of
LS&S, LLC]

Ringer Audible Telephone Signaler TR100

alerts you to your telephone ringing by automatically sounding a loud adjustable horn. It can flash lights and sound horns in other rooms by use of remote receivers. It has adjustable volume and tone controls and requires no batteries (powered by the telephone line). It comes with a five-year factory warranty.

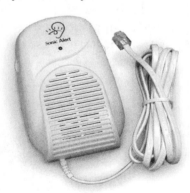

[Photo Courtesy of Adco
Hearing Products, Inc.]

Earware Cell Phone "Hands-Free" Amplifier

plugs into the earphone jack on a cell phone and offers two selectable levels of audio boost with improved listening in background noise. It's ideal for molded earpieces or special headsets that require more volume to oversome the increased air space between the transducer and the eardrum.

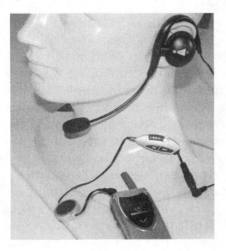

[Photo Courtesy of Harris Communications, Inc.]

Cell-U-Hear Listening Pads

are spongy oval pads that adhere to any cell phone handset enabling improved volume and comfort between your cell phone and your hearing aid. Through its design, it directs sound into the hearing aid for an increase in volume without feedback. The set includes two different ring sizes.

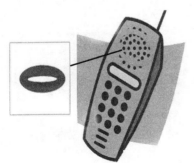

[Photo Courtesy of Harris Communications, Inc.]

Television

DirectEar 100 Personal Listening System
is an infrared wireless system that provides the listener with complete, private and substantial audio amplification (up to 124 dB SPL) of the television, VCR, or compatible audio source, independent of the volume on the set itself. Therefore, it doesn't interfere with other people viewing or listening in the same room. It's also compatible with many infrared amplifying systems in movie theaters and other facilities. In fact, many theaters will allow you to bring the headset with you. The system comes with one rechargeable battery. However, a second rechargeable battery is recommended so that you won't be inconvenienced from listening due to battery recharge time. Operating time is about 10 hours; recharge time is about 14 hours (typically overnight if you use only one battery). The earphone is lightweight. Among several optional accessories, an external microphone for TVs with no audio output capability, and induction neckloop systems compatible with this product are available. It comes with a two-year warranty.

DirectEar 250 Personal Listening System
is quite similar to the system 100 but it cannot be used in movie theaters. One advantage over the 100 system is that the transmitter can charge two batteries at the same time. However, operating time is less, about 6 hours per rechargeable battery.

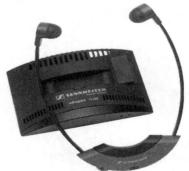

[Photo Courtesy of Hitec Group International, Inc.]

APPENDIX II
Professional Resources

There are a number of service organizations that offer information to consumers with hearing loss. Some offer leaflets or brochures and others offer referral services. Some do not have any current consumer services but are cited here to allow you to write them regarding any questions you might have about a particular problem that you feel might best be addressed by them. Hopefully, this will give you the opportunity to expand your present search.

In the organization listings, in addition to telephone and fax, you should note that all telephone contacts are *voice* unless otherwise specified as TTY (for deaf callers). If you have access to the Internet, you can reach many groups directly through their websites or E-mails. Listings in this section without E-mails can generally be found by directly visiting an organization's website.

In the text that follows, background, company function, and their publications are included. If you're writing a request for information, you're encouraged to enclose a self-addressed, stamped (business-size) envelope, large enough to accommodate the requested literature. If you are telephoning, keep in mind that many of these offices are in the east (EST zone) and some close earlier than 5:00 p.m.

Academy of Dispensing Audiologists

3008 Millwood Avenue, Columbia, SC 29205
Toll Free: (800) 445-8629 Fax: (803) 765-0860
E-mail: info@audiologist.org   Website: www.audiologist.org

Founded in 1977, the Academy supports audiologists who dispense hearing aids. They must have achieved a graduate degree in the field, and in the near future, the only acceptable degree for membership qualification will be a doctorate. The Academy holds an annual meeting in the fall, and during the year smaller regional meetings and seminars providing information regarding all aspects of hearing aid dispensing. *Feedback* is their quarterly magazine for professionals that addresses topics and current issues pertinent to audiologists dispensing hearing aids. As of this writing, they are not staffed for consumer outreach although they offer consumer brochures and professional referrals to a practitioner in your local area.

Alexander Graham Bell Association for the Deaf

3417 Volta Place NW, Washington, D.C. 20007-2770
Tel: (202) 337-5220   TTY: (202) 337-5221   Fax: (202) 337-8314
Website: www.agbell.org

The Association is a nonprofit organization comprised of individuals who are hearing impaired, and their parents, professionals, and others. The organization's mission is to empower those with loss of hearing to function independently by promoting universal rights and optimal opportunities. They provide scholarships and awards to students and their families. They publish two periodicals, one research based, the other consumer oriented. There are over 20 chapters in North America, all of which provide leaflets on a range of problems affecting those suffering with hearing loss.

American Academy of Audiology

11730 Plaza America Drive, Suite 300 Reston, VA 20190
Toll Free: (800) 222-2336   Tel: (703) 790-8466   Fax: (703) 790-8631
E-mail: info@audiology.org   Website: www.audiology.org

The Academy is a professional membership organization of audiologists. They have two primary journal publications. *Audiology Today* is a magazine format that deals with a wide variety of topics including clinical activities and hearing research. The *Journal of the American Academy of Audiology* publishes scientific papers of a scholarly nature. The Academy provide audiologists with current practice information and ongoing research knowledge. Their annual national meeting allows clinicians and scientists a forum for exchange and education in the areas of hearing science and hearing aids. They are not staffed for consumer outreach although they offer consumer brochures and professional referrals.

American Academy of Otolaryngology— Head and Neck Surgery, Inc.

One Prince Street, Alexandria, Va 22314
Tel: (703) 836-4444   TTY: (703) 519-1585   Fax (703) 683-5100
Website: www.entnet.org

Founded in 1896 as a medical specialty society, they now have 11,000 physician members who provide medical care and surgery for disorders of the ears, nose, throat, head and neck regions. The primary missions of the Academy are to provide continuing medical education and to represent the interests of the specialty in governmental areas. The Academy publishes about a dozen patient education leaflets on various aspects of hearing loss which are available to the public at no charge. They also will refer you to a local practitioner if you specifically request the "Physicians List."

American Speech-Language-Hearing Association

10801 Rockville Pike, Rockville, Maryland 20852
Toll Free: (800) 638-8255 Tel: (301) 897-5700 Fax: (301) 571-0457
E-mail: actioncenterwebsite.org   Website: www.asha.org

ASHA is a national professional and scientific association for audiologists and speech-language pathologists. Their mission is to ensure that all people with speech, language or hearing disorders have access to quality services to help them communicate more effectively. They inform the public about communicative disorders through published materials available by request. They can also provide professional referrals.

American Tinnitus Association

P.O. Box 5, Portland, OR 97207
Toll Free: (800) 634 8978   Tel: (503) 248-9985   Fax: (503) 248-0024
E-mail:tinnitus@ata.otg   Website: www.ata.org

This nonprofit organization is dedicated to the support of scientific research leading to a better understanding of tinnitus. They provide pamphlets of information on tinnitus and publish a consumer-based quarterly magazine (by subscription) discussing various issues pertaining to understanding this problem.

The Audiology Awareness Campaign

822 Montgomery Avenue, Suite 318, Narberth, PA 19072
Toll Free: (800) 445-8629   Toll Free (for free literature): (888) 833-3277
www.audiologyawarness.com

AAC was organized by five professional audiology organizations with one goal in mind—helping people with hearing loss. At the website you can take an online "hearing test," read patient-friendly brochures on hearing loss and hearing aids, find out what an audiologist is, post a question on the "Question and Answer" board, and even find an audiologist in your area who can further answer your questions and offer you help. Their web page is one part of the informational process. AAC distributes educational information through various aspects of national media such as newspapers, magazines and television.

Better Hearing Institute

515 King St., Suite 420, Alexandria, VA 22314
Toll Free:(888) 432-7435 Tel: (703) 684-3391 Fax: (703) 684-6048
E-mail:mail@betterhearing.org   Website: www.betterhearing.org

BHI, a nonprofit educational organization, implements public information programs on hearing loss and available hearing solutions for millions with uncorrected hearing loss. The Institute promotes awareness of hearing loss and help through television, radio, and print media public service messages that typically feature well known celebrities who themselves suffer from impaired hearing. You may contact them for literature on hearing loss or specific subjects such as tinnitus, hearing aids, children's ear conditions, lists of local hearing professionals, and assistive listening devices.

The Deafness Research Foundation

1050 17th Street, NW, Suite 701, Washington, DC 20036
Tel: (202) 289-5850   Fax: (202) 293-1805
Website: www.drf.org

Founded in 1958, DFR is a leading source of private funding for basic and clinical research in hearing science. The DRF is committed to making lifelong hearing health a national priority by funding research and implementing education projects in both the government and private sectors. They annually award grants to promising young researchers and established researchers to explore new avenues of hearing science, having awarded over $21 million through more than 1,750 research grants. This seed money has led to dramatic innovations that increase options for those living with hearing loss, as well as protect those at risk. These innovations include the diagnosis and treatment of otitis media (middle ear infections), the cochlear implant, implantable hearing aids, breakthroughs in molecular biology and hair cell regeneration.

Education and Auditory Research Foundation

1817 Patterson St., Nashville, TN 37203
Toll Free: (800) 545-4327 Tel: (615) 627-2724 Fax: (615) 627-2728
E-mail: ear@earfoundation.org   Website: www.earfoundation.org

One of the mission's of the EAR Foundation is to administer education about Meniere's disease through their "Meniere's Network." This is a national network of people who share coping strategies regarding this condition. EAR publishes a few in-depth management brochures which provide education on Meniere's, including dietary management. They also publish a Newsletter, *Steady*, covering many aspects of the problems with Meniere's along with coping strategies. They also publish a Newsletter, *Otoscope*, that addresses problems more associated with hearing loss. They have a *Young Ears* focus on children who suffer from hearing loss, with a helpful section on early detection (what you can expect in normal developmental sounds in the first 24 months of your infant).

Hearing Education and Awareness for Rockers [HEAR] San Francisco Center on Deafness

P.O. Box 460847, San Francisco, CA 94146
Tel: (415) 409-3277 24 Hr Hotline: (415) 773-9590 Fax: (415) 409-5683
E-mail:hear@hearnet.com   Website: www.hearnet.com

HEAR is a nonprofit public-benefit health organization founded in 1988 by Kathy Peck and Flash Gordon, M.D. They inspired large numbers of musicians and medically concerned physicians, music lovers and other music professionals to participate with them. Their advisory board consists of some members—now hearing impaired—from a variety of the loudest 1960's Rock 'n Roll bands. The organization is dedicated to raising consumer awareness about the risks of noise, and its damaging effects on hearing. They achieve this through television and radio public service messages featuring well known artists. Also, they have outreach programs which distribute hearing information and earplugs at music concerts/conferences, health fairs and community events. You may contact them for a free leaflet about noise risks. They've also produced a video on this subject for use in schools.

Hearing Health Magazine

Voice International Publications, Inc.,
P.O. Drawer V, Ingleside, TX 78362-0500
Tel/TTY: (361) 776-7240   Fax: (361) 776-3278
E-mail:ears2u@hearinghealthmag.com
Website: www.hearinghealthmag.com

Owned by the Deafness Research Foundation, Hearing Health's mission is to educate (and entertain) people who are deaf and hard of hearing. Each quarterly issue includes articles ranging from technological research and development, to humor, human success stories, and philosophical discussions about topics like education, cochlear implants, modes of communication, and living without hearing. Contact them for a complimentary current magazine.

International Hearing Society

16880 Middlebelt Rd., Suite 4, Livonia, MI 48154
Toll Free: (800) 521-5247 Tel: (734) 522-7200 Fax (734) 522-0200
Website: www.ihsinfo.org

The IHS began in 1951 as the primary organization for hearing aid dispensers. They conduct programs of competence qualification and training, and offer continuing education courses in the selection, fitting, counseling, and dispensing of hearing instruments. They also publish an industry magazine, the *Audecibel*, articles of which cover issues pertaining to hearing loss and hearing aid electronics, performance and use. A charitable subgroup of the IHS is the Hearing Aid Foundation which specifically focuses on education of the consumer. For a dispenser in your area, you may contact them.

National Institute on Aging - Information Center

P.O. Box 8057, Gaithersburg, MD 20898-8057
Toll Free: (800) 222-2225   TTY: (800) 222-4225   Fax (301) 589-3014
E-mail: niaicjbs1.com   www.nih.gov/nia.

The NIA is responsible for the conduct and support of biomedical, social, and behavioral research, training, health information dissemination, and other programs with respect to the aging process and the diseases and other special problems and needs of the aged. They publish a number of detailed leaflets covering such broad areas as aging, grants, diseases, prevention, medical care, medications, planning for later years, and safety.

National Institute on Deafness and Other Communication Disorders [NIDCD] - Information Clearinghouse

1 Communication Avenue, Bethesda, MD 20892-3456
Tel: (800) 241-1044   TTY: (800) 241-1055   Fax (301) 770-8977
E-mail:nidcdinfo@nidcd.nih.gov   Website: www.nidcd.nih.gov

This is a branch of the U.S. Government's National Institutes of Health. They are an information clearinghouse that provides information on hearing, balance, smell, taste, voice, speech and language disorders. They collect and disseminate information; maintain a computerized database; and develop and distribute publications that include fact sheets, bibliographies, information packets and directories of information resources. The Clearinghouse also publishes a biannual newsletter.

Self Help for Hard of Hearing People, Inc.

7910 Woodmont Avenue, Suite 1200, Bethesda, MD 20814
Tel: (301) 657-2248   TTY: (301) 657-2249   Fax (301) 913-9413
E-mail:national@shhh.org   Website: www.shhh.org

SHHH seeks to provide information and educational outreach to people with hearing loss. Founded in 1979, their membership of 12,000 is the largest consumer organization in the world. Their extensive volunteer-based network includes 250 groups and chapters which reach an additional 9,500 hard of hearing people, their family members, friends, and others. They are governed by a 21-member volunteer board of trustees. SHHH provides its educational offerings in a number of ways, including written materials such as the bimonthly magazine, *Hearing Loss: The Journal of Self Help for Hard of Hearing People*, and other publications and videos; annual conventions for consumers that exceeds 1,000 attendees; encouragement and participation in research activities with the government, private sector, and other nonprofit organizations; and the provision of guidance to national, state and local policy makers and private companies on a wide range of topics affecting people with hearing loss.

INDEX

A

Academy of Dispensing Audiologists, 237
Acoustic Neuroma Association, 238
aging (see *hearing*)
Alexander Graham Bell Assn. for the Deaf, 238
American Academy of Audiology, 238
American Academy of Otolaryngology-Head and Neck Surgery, 238-239
American Speech-Language-Hearing Association, 239
American Tinnitus Association, 239
arteries, hardening of, 134
Assistive Listening Devices, 222-236
audiograms, 43-61, 97
　air, 43-46
　bone, 53
　components of, 43
　frequencies on, 44-61
　mixed loss on, 53
　noise notch on, 51
　pure tones on, 43-49
　speech on, 49-50, 58-59
　thresholds on, 45-61
　whole story not, 61
auditory deprivation, 13-14
auditory training, 214-217
audiologists, 26-31
　background check for, 36
　checkups by, 178
　compassion by, 34

　dependability of, 35
　empathy by, 34
　expectations of, 31
　finding, 31
　level of knowledge of, 33
　likeability of, 34
　temperament of, 34
　trust in, 113
　years of service for, 33
audiology, history of, 27-28

B

batteries (also see *hearing aids*)
　anticipating dead, 155
　conserving, 158
　dead, 154
　defective, 154, 159
　dirty contacts for, 170
　earwax obstruction with, 159
　getting most out of, 155
　short life of, 168
　spent, 157
　stockpiling, 158
　swallowing, 149-150
Battery Ingestion Hotline, 149-150
Better Hearing Institute, 240
brain, reeducating the, 206

C

cardiovascular fitness, 132
cerumen, 97, 144-145
　feedback caused by, 174
　preventing build-up, 160
　removing, 161-162
　responsibility for, 160-162
change, 7, 12, 20

cochlear implants, 145-147
communication strategies,
   200-221
   acknowledgement, 201
   assertiveness, 202
   repair, 214
   tenacity, 203

D

**Deafness Research
   Foundation,** 240
diabetes, 55
dizziness (see *Meniere's
   Disease*), 140-144, 145
drainage from ear, 144
dysequilibrium, 141

E

ear pain, 145
earwax (see *cerumen*)
**Education and Auditory
   Research Foundation,** 241
ego, 5
emotions of losing hearing,
   3-22 (also see *feelings*)
Eustachian tubes, 185-186
exercise and hearing, 132
expectations, 20-21

F

family doctor (see *physicians*)
feedback (see *hearing aids*)
feelings of,
   acceptance, 22
   anger, 14, 16, 63, 74, 114
   anxiety, 14-15, 71, 74-75,
      112, 114
   arrogance, 71

avoidance, 14
   social activities, 63
confusion, 14, 71
defeat, 17-18
defense, 4
depression, 14-15, 20, 63, 70,
   74-75, 112, 114
discontentment, 14, 70
discouragement, 5
disorientation, 4, 14, 71
embarrassment, 19, 63, 87
extroversion, 114
fatigue, 63
fear, 14
frustration, 14, 17-18, 74,
   114
handicap, 87, 127
inadequacy, 4
inattention, 71
incompetence, 4
independence, 71
inferiority, 14
insecurity, 14, 70, 112
instability, 14, 70
intolerance to social
   interaction, 13
irritability, 14, 63
isolation, 14-15, 63, 75, 112
loneliness, 63
looking older with hearing
   aids, 127
negativism, 63, 70
nervousness, 14, 70, 87
paranoia, 14, 71, 74, 114
phobias, 14, 71, 74-75, 114
poor-
   concentration, 14, 71
   health, 63
   job effectiveness, 63
   memory, 63

psychological health, 63
speech recognition, 14
priced out of the market, 114
rejection, 19, 63
resentment, 17
safety,
danger to, 63, 70
self-criticism, 14, 71, 74
self-defeat, 18
self-esteem, 75, 114
selfishness, 17
sensory deprivation, 13-14
stress, 63
temperamental, 14, 70
tension, 14, 63, 70
upset, 87
withdrawal, 75, 192
Food and Drug
Administration, 144

H

hair cell regeneration, 137-
138
hearing,
aerobic exercise and, 133
age-related changes, 182
aging and, 126, 181-199
background noise and, 5
cholesterol and, 133
evaluation, of 38-39
exercise and, 132
expectations and, 20-21
high blood pressure and, 132
human sense of, 4
importance of, 112
influences that affect, 186-
188
miscommunication and, 5
normal, 94, 127
nutrition and, 132-136

poor attention and, 4
smoking and, 132
speechreading and (also see
speechreading), 210-212
stress and, 132
tactics, 217-218
advance planning, 219
microphone technique, 220
move closer, 218
quiet the room, 218
triglycerides and, 133
vitamins and, 135
hearing aids,
adjusting to, 110, 203-204
advantages of BTE/FM, 91
age of your, 117
amplifiers on, 98
analog (see *linear*)
attitudes about, 25
background noises wearing,
105, 122, 124, 177, 185
balanced hearing with, 123
barrel-sounding, 119
batteries in (also see
batteries), 98, 100
in backwards in, 156
dirty contacts, 170
battery ingestion, 149-150
Behind-The-Ear (BTE), 96-
97, 99, 168
benefits of, 72-75, 125
brain and, 121
candidacy for, 83-84, 94-95
comfort with, 101
Completely-In-Canal (CIC),
19, 83, 95, 99, 113, 119-
120
advantages of, 100
disadvantages of, 100
controls on your, 118
cosmetically appealing, 111

P

physicians, 37, 76, 125-127, 144
pistols, 187
prejudices (see *hearing aids* and *hearing loss*)
professional help, seeking, 23-42
professional resources, 237-243

Q

quality of life, 62-77

R

rifles, 187

S

Self Help for Hard of Hearing People, Inc., 243
sensory deprivation, 12-13
sensory stimulation, 13
shotguns, 187
significant others (also see *spouses*), 20-21, 31, 179-180
speechreading, 206-214
   familiarity with the language, 209
   principles of, 207-214
   restricting lip movements, 208-209
   topic restrictions, 209-210
   visibility of, 207-208
speech recognition, 14
spouses (also see *significant other*), 20-21

T

telecoils (see *hearing aids*)
telephone use (see *hearing aids*)
television,
   assistive listening, 148
   too loud, 6
tinnitus, 123

U

U.S. Surgeon General, 132

V

vents (see *hearing aids*)
vertigo, 140-144
vestibular compensation, 141
vestibular neuritis, 141
Veterans Administration, 114
vitamins and hearing, 135

Y

yellow pages, 37